Presence in Solitude

Presence in Solitude

The Pastoral Promise of the Pandemic

ROBERT C. BECKMAN JR.

RESOURCE *Publications* · Eugene, Oregon

PRESENCE IN SOLITUDE
The Pastoral Promise of the Pandemic

Resource Publications
An Imprint of Wipf and Stock Publishers
199 W. 8th Ave., Suite 3
Eugene, OR 97401

www.wipfandstock.com

PAPERBACK ISBN: 978-1-6667-3369-3
HARDCOVER ISBN: 978-1-6667-2857-6
EBOOK ISBN: 978-1-6667-2860-6

SEPTEMBER 28, 2021

Contents

Introduction

THE CLOCKS HAVE STOPPED

December 07, 2020

The Clocks have stopped
but time has not
What then shall we do?

Await the end of what we crave,
Try not to misbehave?

My watch is slowed
time still goes
what then shall we become?

Await the face of what we fear
hold all our loved one's near?

The clocks have stopped
But time has not what then
Shall we pray?

To bend the arc of circumstance
Let kindness show the way?

The clocks have stopped
But time has not how long
Oh Lord to wait?

Until the Son of Man appears
As your neighbor by the way.

"@7.20, COFFEE, PERAMBULATE, PRAYERS." That is generally the first line every morning in my notebook. I write the time I arrive in my study, hang my coat and stow my gear. Going immediately to the kitchen I make the morning coffee. Cafe Bustelo. Three bucks a pop at Dollar General. It is a bold espresso style coffee primarily known as a Hispanic brand despite solid New York City origins. Cafe Bustelo is a brand often associated with Cuban-style coffee. For me, it is "work coffee." I drink it in my study. It is strong and rich, and I take it sweet. I don't think I'm the only one who hopes that rich, sweet coffee will be reflected in my time studying Scripture-that the Word will speak to me rich and sweet.

As the coffee brews I go into the church auditorium[1]. I listen to the same piece of music by the same artist every day. *Spiegel im Spiegel*, composed by Arvo Pärt, as played by Anne Akiko Myers. I walk around the auditorium and read the *Morning Prayers* from the Daily Office published online by the Northumbrian Community. This process from the moment I enter the auditorium takes around 10 minutes. I am generally finished reading and praying before the music stops.

Then, I pour the coffee, go to my study, and continue with the mission. Being a creature of habit, I have pursued a form of this pattern for many years. What was a predisposition became a fully formed ritual in mid-March 2020. It was about this time that society ground to a halt. People were sick. People were afraid. The economy was in shock. Plague and pandemic were things which

---

1. A church house is just a structure until the Body of Christ is present. When the Body is at worship it is a sanctuary. On your typical Thursday it's just an auditorium.

happened to other people living in third-world countries. How, we thought, could this happen to us? Here? Now?

Because I pastor a small church, in a small town, in a far-off, isolated, and nearly forgotten corner of the country, I did not miss a day of work.[2] Even during the large swath of time we have been meeting virtually I made my way to the church house every day. I made my small, coded entry into my notebook; walked, read, listened, prepared my heart, and then studied scripture.

And now, as the world begins to haltingly emerge from a chrysalis season, we have to ask ourselves *"what have we learned, what have we become."* And we must ask even more difficult questions. What have we lost? What have we gained? Do the gains outweigh the losses?

As I write these words we are passing through a second winter hoping against hope for a new kind of spring. A spring which not only promises fresher weather but a fresher Spirit. A season not only of new growth but also of new hope.

But before all of this starts to read like the crawl that opens a *Star Wars* movie let me make some formal acknowledgements:

- Mrs. Beckman, my lovely wife.
- Cafe Bustelo.
- Arvo Pärt/Anne Akiko Myers & Como Audio.
- Field Notes Brand notebooks.
- The *Notorious Edwards County Preachers.* (Dustin, Clayton, Jacob, Lance.)
- The elders and leaders at Grayville First Christian Church.
- My friends and readers. Wes, who knows me, and who always speaks wisely. Wade, who has engineers eyes. Steve, who read the manuscript and suggested "revisiting the title."

---

2. For my wife and me the inside joke was: "In Southeastern Illinois we were already social distancing." Mrs. Beckman is a little anti-social. For her the jubilant quote was "I've been preparing for this my whole life."

- Additional thanks are due to Logos Bible Software and Accordance Bible Software.

Prologue

EVERY DAY I LEAVE the Parsonage on the Hill, the woman I love, a place of domestic comfort to do the work of ministry. Every day-every single day-that work of ministry is subtly different. This has never been more true than during our quarantine season. Interventions I would have unthinkingly made 18 months ago are simply not possible. Pastoral calls. Sitting at the Hospital. Serendipitously bumping into church members at a restaurant. Attending high school and Jr High sports, concerts, plays, sales, and carnivals. Many if not most of those things have simply stopped. Like everyone else I have had to change my approach to work. I have had to learn how to increase the reach of ministry while wearing restraints. I have had to learn how to preach the gospel without people present. Guys like me have had to learn how to be producers and content creators so that we might stream worship online and provide fresh content for new communication mediums. We have had to become even more capable of using the telephone, text, chat, and Zoom-not as useful adjuncts to "real ministry" but as essential tools. It has been exhausting, exhilarating, and expansive. It will come to an end. Soon, I hope. But if it does not ministry will continue. (As I write these very words, I know that within the next 45 minutes I will jump on Facebook Live to read scripture and provide a simple touch to folk who have been in "the cave".)

Yes, it will end. What of the journey? Why has this happened? Who are you now? Have you moved forward or regressed? How have you coped? When will "normal", "new-normal", "alternative normal", finally happen? When we drill down using the central interrogatories of human inquiry, we find ourselves in that strange place where asking questions does not generate answers but only leads to more questions. If we have gone through this long challenging year and nothing has changed, we have wasted an opportunity which may never come in quite the same way again.

1

We are not the first. We will not be the last. And right now, you are not the only. Let that sink in. In the twenty-first century, in the developed world, in an advanced country, we tend to define ourselves as much on our feelings of superiority and uniqueness if not more than we rely on our faith. As a preacher it is my vocation to mine the scriptures, not only for comforting mottos to trot out at difficult times, but to expose from the Word of God the vast treasures which help to contextualize and make sense of our common human experience. Because I believe the Bible to be the true, inspired, and authoritative Word of God I expect the Church to not only be informed by the Bible but to be formed by it. It breaks my heart when Christian people think of themselves as immune from the environmental flotsam and jetsam which circulates in the world. Our faith was born in a specific act of illegal, unreasonable violence. Yet, it turned out OK. Reading the Bible is not, or at least should not, be a means for finding exceptions to the basic rules of reality. The promise of God's strengthening presence to lift us up is pointless if we always pray that we never find ourselves down. The indwelling Holy Spirit is superfluous if "we've got this." Why pray for strength when we wish to never be weak? We ask for deliverance because we crave comfort and prefer safety. What's the point of resurrection if we do not wake every morning with the aches and pains which are practical reminders of mortality? The love we share with our spouses should prepare us and ennoble us for the love between Jesus and His called, yet (seemingly) perpetually imperfect Bride. He is making Her ready for the wedding day-even if it takes all eternity. Literally.

For us then, the Bible must be many things. A book of many dimensions, many colors. For us the Bible is (should be . . . must be) art, architecture, arc. It provides structure and strategy, doctrine and practice, sight, and insight. It not only helps the Church to know but also to do. Whilst non-christians may not agree with nor be obedient to the Bible, my Christian "worldview" instructs me that the truths revealed in the Bible are still applicable to all humans. Like the mathematical certainty of physics and the mysterious machinations of love, you don't have to agree with it to be subject to and described by it. Truth is not susceptible to assent.

So, in turning to the Bible.

- To "understand life".
- To "make sense of it."
- To "get a grip".

As human beings in general and the Church in particular, we are constantly looking for information, inspiration, and insight. And the Bible delivers. Are we wise enough, are we disciplined enough, are we discerning enough to hear what the Bible is saying and to properly apply what it teaches to our new, emerging, troubling, and challenging circumstances?

That is our premise. That is our starting point. What else could it be? Kingdom broke into the world some twenty-one centuries ago and Empire has spent that entire span of time extracting its pound of flesh from the faithful. Answering the question "are you a Christian?" has, for far too many become just another cultural identity marker mainly determined by one's ideological or imperial allegiance. Some christians might sing *This world is not my home, I'm only passing through,* but subsequent behavior betrays their true allegiance. The time seems past when church members thought of themselves as a "third race." History has swallowed the memory of christians who saw in politics the diabolical hand of Empire. Now rather than holding the culture accountable and bringing the Gospel to bear on Empire some have determined that the task of believers is to infiltrate, assimilate, consolidate, and legitimate Empire so that it serves *our* ends. If it changes us and our relationship to Gospel; so be it. We have waited long enough. It is our time. We are different. We are benevolent. We can be trusted. How quickly and completely we forget.

Remember, at different times and in different places the paths and processes of Empire and Kingdom have not only crossed . . . they've often been mixed. The sprawling amalgamation of faith, superstition, heroism, ignorance, brilliance, backwardly looking advancement, retrenchment and innovative antiquarianism called *Christendom* is the prime historic example. Much to admire, much to doubt, much amazement, and at the end, St. Thomas Aquinas. Certainly, God was a part of what Christendom was and what Christendom was becoming, or at least what it was trying to be, but there were also enormous parts of it from which He was absent. Absent by his choice or by expulsion. Expelled by the forces of Empire which rose and fell within Christendom, sometimes holding the levers of power, other times exiled from power, ridiculed, or persecuted. And sadly, at other times locked in a perpetual battle for power.

Through long months of pandemic, the Empire of this world has debated, delegated, bloviated, proclaiming the power to solve a problem which was from the very first beyond the power of Empire to control. When centralizing strategies failed, Empire denigrated, desecrated, and pontificated, creating an entire new vocabulary of moral platitude and human "follyocracy."[1] All, again to seek a solution for a disease which proved blithely apathetic to human intervention. Hopes and prayers were offered by people who were hopeless and faithless because amid crisis the spiritual nature at the core of humanity peeks out of society's feckless sheath and begs for mercy from the very God whose existence is relentlessly denied by Empire's power.

And yet I am hopeful. Not for hope's sake but for God's sake. I am hopeful because where Empire fails Kingdom prevails. When

---

1 Follyocracy; Noun. The bureaucratization of foolishness.

Empire retreats, Kingdom revives. When Empire is at its worst it is then that Kingdom is at its very best. When Empire sees only death, the culture of death, the stench of death, the despair of death, it is then, and it is there that Kingdom sees life.

So as a believer and as a preacher, which is to say as someone who tells and retells the story of Jesus, I am convinced that God's Word addresses the very questions advanced by a weary society and worried Church. Individually and collectively human society has gone through this before. The Church has addressed circumstances like this before. God's people have not only weathered storms like this-maybe worse than this-but while we were weathering these past "storms of the century" God's people went about sheltering, clothing, feeding, comforting, and caring for those who did not share our love for Jesus but who did share our humanity. By loving and serving those who did not yet call upon the name of Jesus we, by our actions, proclaimed the veracity of the inspired words we preached.

This is my call to the Church to be the Church in desperate times. It is beyond time for us to complain about circumstances. Rather, it is time to creatively address these new realities-these new opportunities-which are emerging in a post-pandemic world. Because I am a preacher I will deal with scripture. We will examine some Biblical stories which help us to deal with the questions: "what has this all been for? What has the isolation gifted me? Have I changed? How can Jesus use me better? Or, having succumbed to selfishness do I simply crawl back into the hole and give in to the temptations of blame, shame, fear, fatigue, and apathy?"

In pursuing these deep, sometimes existential questions I must clarify what this journey will not do, where it will not go, what it will not be.

- Political
- Economic
- Sociological
- Psychological

Each of these dimensions of human understanding has played a significant role in the unfolding of our quarantine season. For some, focusing on these issues has become the obsessive driver of discontent, discouragement, despair, and denunciation. I fear that if we continue along the current path, both church and society will find that these short-sighted answers to our current quandaries will also result in damnation. You cannot build the kingdom of heaven with bricks first used in the building of Babel. And it is time for the church to quit it. Just stop. Knock it off. If you want to play politics, resign your pulpit, study poly-sci, and run for office. If you want to reduce it all to money and make mammon your God—you can, but you must realize that you have been forewarned. If you want to fight it out on the field of social/psychological/anthropological/ mythological/alchemical nonsense; have at it, God bless you but leave me out of it. None of that stuff is working and it is time for the Church of Jesus Christ to get out of the business of peddling the impotent snakeoil of others and get back into the business of telling the old, old, story of Jesus and His love.

To some this might seem overly simplistic, even naive. Others, would say, much more directly, that this is a stupid approach. Not so. Let me remind you of what happened to the Apostle Paul when he sought to approach the cultured elites of his day with the arguments *of* the cultured elites. It is amazing how easy it is to forget the Biblical stories which are most applicable to a particular situation, which deal with the very issues we face.

Paul makes his way to Athens. He is summoned to the central shrine, of the leading city of the Hellenistic ethos. It was the epitome of modern[2] cultured society in the first century. In Athens, the university educated, politically astute, and the philosophically sophisticated citizens held endless seminars regarding the latest Epicurean and Stoic sophistries which were guaranteed to

2. Like "contemporary" as a description of music, cinema, worship styles and etc. we have to be careful of using the word Modern as a modifier based upon our (Modern) way of thinking. Modern and contemporary first and foremost describe what is going on NOW, whenever NOW is located in time and space. When Paul was there Athens was modern, PostModern, with-it Avant-garde.

expand the empire, enlarge the treasury, and extend the reputation of Athenian learning. You could ask them and they would gladly tell you that was exactly what was going on. Paul came to them speaking of a resurrected Jesus and they mistakenly thought he was talking about two Gods. He was asked to come clarify this new, strange, ticklish tidbit of knowledge and he gladly accepted their invitation.

He talked about God the creator. He spoke of God's patience with human frailty and folly. He illustrated and colored his message with quotations from the extensive store of their own philosophical and poetic knowledge. He addressed Hellenistic spirituality as somewhat ignorant but due to neither malice or simplicity. He introduced Jesus as God's representative and Judge validated by His resurrection from the dead . . . and they laughed. All cultured Greeks were believers in the eternality of the soul, some embracing soul-migration or reincarnation. They curtly dismissed him and only a few believed.

> *"Acts 17:32 Now when they heard of the resurrection of the dead, some mocked. But others said, "We will hear you again about this." Acts 17:33 So Paul went out from their midst. Acts 17:34 But some men joined him and believed, among whom also were Dionysius the Areopagite and a woman named Damaris and others with them." (Acts 17:32–34 ESV)*

Later, as Paul continued his ministry though the various cities and regions of the Hellenized world, he determined that a full-fledged adaptation of the cultural, literary, rhetorical, and philosophical tools available within Hellenism was inappropriate to telling the story of Jesus. We must understand culture to address it but not be enslaved by its assumptions, models, or methods. While Paul was always contextualizing and molding the message to his audience, he anchored the project fully to the scriptures. For Paul that required the hard work of exegeting culture alongside his exegesis of scripture. Writing to the Corinthians he reminded them how he came to them proclaiming the empowering foolishness of the cross.

So also, when I came to you brothers, I did not come trying to demystify the message by *cloaking* it in a *culturally-
conditioned rhetorical flourish*. Nope. Instead, I decided
to know nothing amongst you rather than the story of
Jesus the crucified.[3]

Now, Paul was no dummy and there are clearly times
throughout his preaching and writing career that he was perfectly
capable of understanding and quoting from the culturally acceptable sources of knowledge of his day. However, after Athens
he chose to not do in Rome as they do in Rome, not because he
couldn't but because that was not his job and the story the culture
was telling was not his story. Perhaps we need to be reminded now
and again of how Paul approached telling the story of Jesus in the
context of cultural rejection.

For too long we have mixed the business of the Kingdom
with the things of earth. We have polluted the story of the cross,
watering it down with the strategies of Empire. No wonder the
world laughs at the Church. Our Kingdom words are drowned
out by the imperial tone we too often take. It is not naive, foolish,
short-sighted, or stupid to leave behind the cultural flourishes of
power, prestige, political resonance, and partisan gamesmanship
to know and proclaim only the message of the Cross. To unasham-
edly proclaim the culturally abhorrent message of a humiliated
and crucified Savior is the proper preparation for proclaiming the
triumphant resurrection of the Son of God.

Make no mistake. They may have laughed in Athens, jeered
in Jerusalem, giggled in Galatia and ROFL'd in Rome.[4] But they
were all afraid. They were terrified of this defiantly confident group
which resigned from the pursuit of power. For, in choosing not
to contend for power, first Jesus, and then the earliest Church
disarmed the Empire and prevented it from playing the game it

3. this is our first "Bobslation" in this project. It is a translation/paraphrase
of a NT citation designed to amplify and contemporize a text to which, you
have become inoculated because of mundane familiarity.

4. Jesus!? The guy that half-wit incompetent Pilate killed? GOD? Resurrected. You. Must. Be. Joking?!

played best. When Jesus admitted powerlessness, intimidation failed. When Jesus stated that His Kingdom was not of this world, the temptations of this world lost their bite. When Jesus, Stephen, James, Paul, (the other) James, and countless multitudes who followed, failed to flinch at whip, cross, flame, or sword: that robbed the Empire of the ultimate punishment. You cannot deprive someone of life whose hope is held in the nail-scarred hands of one who has harrowed hell itself.

2

Let's talk about the archaeology of this book. The purpose for which I am writing, and the process I am implementing is to tell Biblical stories of real or perceived isolation so that we might not only be encouraged and comforted in our own time of quarantine but so that we might find applicable guidance and direction for how we should proceed going forward.

Telling Biblical stories can be done at a variety of levels of complexity. As a pastor-theologian-preacher it is my joy and responsibility to tell these stories in a variety of different contexts throughout the typical year-sometimes throughout the typical day.

When preparing to preach, my favored communication model is read/exegete/proclaim. It is a formal model of enduring historical precedent intended to provide information and direction to the Church. This is the means by which the spiritual formation of God's people has been accomplished for generations. There are times, however, when the audience is not old enough or is in some other way unable to process any complex or abstract information, much less Biblical. Children. The Elderly, the intellectually challenged-each of these groups need to hear and can hear the stories of Jesus communicated in such a way that they can *have ears to hear*. People who are incarcerated, incapacitated, institutionalized or hospitalized-being in a different context will need to have the story told in such a way that it speaks to that specific context.

My approach here is not purely exegetical nor fully expositional. It is not mere reading for readings sake. My goal is to take you on a reflective journey into some well known Biblical stories investigating and experiencing what can be taught about isolation. Prison. Desert. Garden. Cross. Exile. These were, for the individuals experiencing them, a kind of social distancing. A time apart. A separation. Through probing their experience and peeking into their solitude we can learn valuable lessons. We can learn how people of faith can thrive through adversity. We should learn that adversity is often only as adverse as we want to make it. We can observe that in loneliness we may find an irreplaceable opportunity to fellowship with God. In short, we can find the presence of God in solitude. In engaging with their time of testing it can help us to correctly process and learn the right lessons from what has become a memorable and sometimes terrifying year.

It will pass. The gates will be unhitched. The doors will swing wide open. Things *will* open up. There is going to be an after. There is going to be a "what's next" and I fear that we will not be ready. I fear that we will not have learned a thing. I fear that we will look back on this year and as we contemplate God's *Presence* in our *Solitude* we will try and claim a victory we have not earned because we have spent so much time complaining, that we have not engaged in the struggle to which we should have been committed. At times I fear that we have expected far too little of the Church and coddled far too much. We have comforted people who have suffered no real loss. True, there are many who have buried loved ones taken by this disease. There are many whose careers have been destroyed. There is real economic despair and exhaustion with demagoguery. Yet there are times when we have focused on what hurts the least, simply so that we might feel better.

Many, inside the Church and out, have reacted with shallow resentment that a harsh reality failed to respect the boundaries of privilege which they had used as a barrier against every sort of undesirable thought or experience. There are fundamental questions about the nature of the Gospel and the purpose of the Church which we need to answer. Right now, I am afraid. If the questions were put to us, we would be insulted by or ignorant of the correct questions and the concrete, Biblical answers. Have we grown closer to God? Has our faith deepened? Have we recommitted to the lessons of faithless, selfless service taught by Jesus? Are we ready to serve our world as the isolation ends? It is not the job of the Church to make you happy. It is not the job of the Church to make you comfortable. It is not the job of the Church to help you "find yourself." If is not the job of the Church to exile the monsters you might have hiding beneath your bed. The time for comforting pats on the back is past. It's time for the Church to raise its expectations and start kicking the lazy, the complacent, and the narcissistic in the tail. We need to remind ourselves again and again, the job of the Church is not to merely enable people to survive bad circumstances

> "Him we proclaim, warning everyone and teaching everyone with all wisdom, that we may present everyone mature in Christ." (Colossians 1:28 ESV)

This proclaiming, warning, and teaching that Paul is talking about is not a strategy for mere survival. It is a strategy for growth. It is a strategy for maturity. It is a strategy for thriving.

In short, it is time for adult Christians to act like it. Put on real pants! Open the curtains! Shower, shave and, shape up! You are called by a forward-thinking Savior to proclaim a message of hope and reconciliation to a lost and discouraged world.

To do this we will look to the scriptures for analogous situations. Let me be clear. We are looking at these stories as analogous- not the same. The world is different. Experiences change. Culture is always shifting. In applying scripture, we are always aligning the horizon of the past with the horizon of the present. That's how it works. The stories we will examine are about individuals going through a similar time of testing or isolation as what we have experienced during the pandemic. Fortunately, we can learn from similarly situated individuals whose example of faithful interaction with God informs ours. In a sense this is what all effective preaching and teaching of narrative Biblical texts does. It uses example, comparison, evocation, parallels, and contextualization to bridge the gap between the ancient text and our modern world.

Unfortunately, far too much preaching and teaching does nothing more than draw (often improper) moral conclusions from the text, using those conclusions to construct morality tales far removed from the intent of the Biblical author(s). We do not need any more prosaic morality tales. We need to look at Biblical characters who confronted isolation, loneliness, separation, or "social distancing" with a view to our own growth and maturity throughout the entire experience. We need to see how these individuals dealt with all the emotional baggage that attends these sorts of circumstances. Despair. Anxiety. Depression. Are these emotional reactions to circumstances inevitable or are there strategies available which disciples can employ which help us to grow and thrive in difficult circumstances? Do our songs sung in solitude have to be dirges, or can we dance a jig?

In moving toward an answer to that last question let's get back to structure and stories and strategy. In the scriptures, there are stories-some very familiar-in which the primary character(s) find themselves in a "quarantine" situation. Either by God's design, their own decision, or the destructive behaviors of others. They are isolated from others, cast upon their own spiritual resources, reduced to a complete dependence upon God. We will look at stories in which the protagonist must live by faith in a difficult and demanding context. It is not exactly like quarantine. It was not called social distancing. Again, we learn and apply scripture by analogy. Not everything we learn from in the Bible is a proposition. Sometimes we learn from understanding narrative structure and by identifying with the Biblical hero we read about. Sometimes God really wants us to figure things out rather than needing to codify our responses. We read of no stone tablets in the New Testament. We do, however, read lots of stories from which Jesus and His inspired Apostles expect us to draw our own conclusions.

So, we will look at the following: Jesus in the wilderness. Jesus in the Garden. Jesus on the Cross. Paul (and Silas) in prison in Philippi. John on Patmos. Each of these individuals are emblematic of how a faithful person should respond to quarantine, isolation, loneliness, forced separation.

1

Desert and Scripture

I asked for water.
I got sand.
This was not the retreat
I had planned.

I hoped to spend some time
In prayer
Somehow Satan
Found me there.

I forgot the snacks
The sunscreen too
My phone is dead
What should I do?

Out of the menacing
Mirage in my head
I heard a voice
Here's what it said:

All that you need
What you want, what you see . . .
It can be yours
If you just bow to me!

I shook off the cobwebs
I opened my eyes
And there I saw Jesus
To my surprise

"Don't mind him friend,
His temptation's a sham . . .
He tried it with me
And you know . . . who . . . I AM"

A FAMILIAR STORY

IN ONE WAY OR another all three synoptic gospels repeat what must have been a familiar and empowering story of the temptation of Jesus. Answering the question as to why it was empowering (He is after all, the Son of God) likely goes a long way towards explaining why it was interesting enough to be repeated to the different Gospel audiences.

The passing of centuries and the literary and editorial stability of the Biblical text is both bane and a blessing. It is a blessing because our generation has been blessed with more versions, explanations, commentaries, summaries, paraphrases, expositions, devotions, and sermons bringing the Bible to light than at any other time in human history. For crying out loud, most Christians (I repeat this an awful lot), for most of Christian history, were illiterate. The only Bible they got was at Church. Only the rich could afford copies of the Bible of their very own and even if you were that rare person of means who could afford a copy of scripture, you had to be able to read for it to have any value to you. So, we who are living in the twenty-first century are blessed with an abundance of materials which make it not only possible to read the Bible but also to engage with tools that contribute to a deeper understanding of what it says. Reading the Bible for us is not only possible, but also culturally permissible, and individually profitable. And even in an increasingly secular and skeptical age it is expected, within most Church traditions, that the Bible will be read, respected, and even appreciated.

This rich blessing with respect to the Biblical text is balanced by the bane I alluded to earlier: we don't tell the story—any stories much anymore. We are too sophisticated for that. Our approach to the Bible whether evangelical, as I am, liberal, or progressive tends toward the formal and forensic. Make no mistake, this approach to studying the Bible is valuable and rewarding and necessary. However, reading the story, understanding the tale, experiencing the yarn, and being embedded in the environment is just as indispensable to comprehending the full revelatory power of God's word. We study the Bible for understanding. We study the Bible to know God through the Word He has inspired and provided. Revelation is seen, heard, felt, smelt, touched, and tasted. It is whispered, it is shouted, it is sung, it is danced it is wept. In short, revelation is a full-blown experience.

So read the Story. Read it deeply. Use all your senses. Access the entire apparatus of understanding through which God discloses Himself to those who earnestly seek Him. As you read this particular story you will need to get into a desert or wilderness frame of mind. Try and taste the dust caked on your tongue. Lick your lips looking for the only liquid relief available, your own increasingly salty sweat. Thinking yourself back into that desolate lonely wilderness helps you to not only read these words but to in some way experience them.[1]

> 1 *Then Jesus was led up by the Spirit into the wilderness to be tempted by the devil. 2 And after fasting forty days and*

---

1. About the NT Biblical text. When I am providing an entire story by paragraph or pericope I will use the English Standard Version. My analysis and exegesis of that text as well as the comments will be based upon my own understanding and translation of the Greek text, generally following the Nestle-Aland 28/UBS 5 text.

forty nights, he was hungry. 3 And the tempter came and said to him, "If you are the Son of God, command these stones to become loaves of bread." 4 But he answered, "It is written, " 'Man shall not live by bread alone, but by every word that comes from the mouth of God.' " 5 Then the devil took him to the holy city and set him on the pinnacle of the temple 6 and said to him, "If you are the Son of God, throw yourself down, for it is written, " 'He will command his angels concerning you,' and " 'On their hands they will bear you up, lest you strike your foot against a stone.' " 7 Jesus said to him, "Again it is written, 'You shall not put the Lord your God to the test.' " 8 Again, the devil took him to a very high mountain and showed him all the kingdoms of the world and their glory. 9 And he said to him, "All these I will give you, if you will fall down and worship me." 10 Then Jesus said to him, "Be gone, Satan! For it is written, " 'You shall worship the Lord your God and him only shall you serve.' " 11 Then the devil left him, and behold, angels came and were ministering to him. Matthew 4:1–11 (ESV)

A Powerful Plot

Matthew knew plot! Perhaps he learned that skill from Jesus. There is evidence in His own story telling process that Jesus was perfectly able and certainly willing to use the power of plot to build suspense and engagement in His audience. There are obvious times when His teaching to our eyes and ears, despite two millennia of advancement and a million years of media evolution, would certainly seem more to us like performance than preaching. Regardless of the nature of the media there is nothing that increases attention, retention, and excitement like plot. And this story, the first one in which Jesus is really the central character[2] has all the elements

2. I would expect some push-back on that statement, but I stand by it. In the Prologue His is just a name. In the infancy narratives His parents, the Magi and even Herod play the central dramatic roles. In the third chapter Jesus makes what would, in a movie, amount to a cameo role and John the Baptist is the star. So, it is here that Jesus emerges as the central character in the story of His life and Gospel.

which make for a great, well-plotted, page turning, hide-behind-the furniture story.

Jesus skillfully and creatively helps us to feel the heat of the sun on our shoulders. Our eyes grow bleary with the desert heat. We lose sense of time and perspective. Hunger gnaws. Thirst thickens. The desert is a place of immense beauty. The creatures who live there are uniquely adapted for the baking, waterless landscape. To people like us, it is these environmental features, these quirks of creation which are the fixtures of deserts most noticeable to us. As creatures who enjoy comforts and easy access to the essential elements we need for survival the mere notion of a place defined by scarcity; regardless of its beauty, fills us with anxiety.

It is true that there are cultures which have thrived in the harshest of desert environments. These cultures tend toward the small, the self-contained or loosely interdependent confederation. Because in a land of scarcity everybody must be satisfied with a little less food and water.

Desert people become comfortable with silence. They are not awed by space. They form a kind of partnership with solitude. In that space, surrounded by the furtive sound of lonely creatures, they come to understand the concept of a creator God with a silent intensity unavailable to those of us who have only envisioned the world through the eyes of verdant civilization in any one of its normative expressions.

One issue which handicaps modern and postmodern people is being unable to find a deserted place, arid or arctic, in mountains or valleys where we might define a definite and distinct conception of what is out there, what has been created, and the creative mind who established it in all of its massive, distributed and diverse glory. We need places where we process life. We need silence. We need to be apart. We need something like a desert retreat where we can have formative experiences which can become a place from which we can view our world and seek to understand eternity

Perhaps that is what frightened and unsettled so many secular, western, cultured individuals when the COVID-19 pandemic drove society apart. We were in places we found familiar. Homes we had selected and decorated with our spouses. Safe spaces defined by all the comforts we constantly crave, all the stuff we strenuously accumulate. Despite the fact we were not going anywhere and in fact did not go anywhere for an inconceivably long time we looked upon these places of domestic joy and tranquility as foreboding places. We saw our own homes as deserts; now unfamiliar because they had been transformed into places of unchosen and unbroken reflection. The people we loved most and held dearest we suddenly saw as either fellow prisoners or possible competitors for what must certainly be limited resources. We chose a home, not the site for a retreat or a recalibration or a rethinking of who we were and what we wanted out of life. We looked our solitude in the face, blinked and wished our experience on someone else, somewhere else, preferably far, far away.

Jesus had surely been in deserted places before. It is hardly possible to move from town to city to village throughout Galilee or Judea or the surrounding jurisdictions without walking through deserted places. What we in the modern world call "the country-side" was always "the wilderness" in that ancient time and place. Farmers did not live on or near their land in homely cottages or even mighty farmhouses. Where Jesus grew to maturity farmers lived in villages. Farmers walked into the countryside to work their fields returning home every evening. Shepherds were only in the field during certain seasons. The whole countryside—everything outside of village or city was rightly thought of as uninhabitable, desolate, wilderness. Goats and constant conflict had transformed what had been a land flowing with milk and honey into a land eroding into an epic past or blowing away in the winds of Empire. The only thing found in deserted wilderness was the jackal, the vulture, and a few other creatures unavailable to the practicing Jew as food.

Jesus chose the wilderness. Driven there, compelled by the Holy Spirit to spend time in prayer, meditation, and preparation for everything that was to come. Jesus chose to remove Himself from what was familiar and comfortable so that in that abandoned wasteland He might find the space He needed to inaugurate the presence of Kingdom. It was said that the Empire made deserts and called it peace. Jesus went to the desert to begin making peace; to define a Kingdom in which authentic peace was won through dutiful, submissive, sacrifice.

Few of us even aspire to such feats of self-resignation and introspection. Few of us in our cultured societies of ease and plenty are willing to be led by the spirit into paths of righteousness— much less paths of personal deprivation so that the righteousness we should crave can be nurtured and grown. If the incarnate Son of God needed to spend time in solitude to prepare for His life's mission perhaps, we should rethink our approach to the formative experience of contemplative, directive, submissive, solitude.

When we look at Jesus' desert experience, we find not only a model to follow but also a singular historical event which impacts all Christian experience. He was in that desert for all of us who now follow Him in faith. He relied on scripture thereby teaching us to rely on scripture. He prayed, instructing us to pray. He resisted the temptations of the evil one, reminding us that Satan will flee us as well when we put up a fight; embedded in prayer and Biblical thinking.

Jesus' experience was formative not only for His ministry but also for how His emissaries would feel when they took His story-formed message to other kinds of deserts. Places where the oracles of God had never been read. Cities and towns where superstition made a mockery of imperial claims to rising modernity. They would take His gospel to lands which had different traditions, different origin myths, strange languages, bizarre cults (theirs always are, ours not so much), odd notions of right and wrong. In short, the nature, the heat, the landscape, the physical threat might change but for the early Church Jesus' story of desert temptation always rang true. Ephesus was just as lonely. Just as deserted. Just as snakey as the Judean Wadi's and hill-country of Jesus' own desert experience.

Geography and landscape and relative temperature change. But spiritual creatures like us need formative experiences. We need experiences where and when we are isolated from all those things, all that stuff which makes it so hard to listen closely and hear the voice of God. He needs us in deserts so that He does not need to shout all the time. He needs us to distance ourselves from the shared commonality of life so that He might teach us about Himself. He needs to teach us by contrasting our smallness with the vast emptiness of the desert. If we cannot handle the terrestrial emptiness of a desert, how could we possibly hope to understand the larger loneliness of the universe?

In wilderness spaces we can clearly differentiate our own yearning from Satan's cleverly concocted visions of community. For in his insatiable desire to divide and conquer Satan is quite efficient at creating communities of divisive sameness and sterile toxicity. He creates chaos in our hearts not to test our character and mold it into the likeness of our Creator but to shatter that bond and turn us against all of God's molding providence.

If we are to make a clear distinction between the small voices with which God whispers and the deafening shout of defiant temptation we must come to grips with isolation and distance and quarantine. It is only lonely if you find it restrictive. It is only a burden if you are unwilling to be molded.

So, God uses Matthew, a former tax-collector, to tell the story of His Son's desert sojourn. His goal is not to amaze or entertain us with Jesus' feat of spiritual gigantism but to reach out through his words, turning back all the intervening years, brushing off the dust, inviting us to participate in His ongoing remaking of the world. After all, before creation, before He spoke into the void, before Logos released the creative impulse upon the face of the deep All was chaos. Wilderness. Barren. Void. Nothing. To summarize: uninhabited wilderness.

Location. Characters. Deprivation. Spiritual, social, and emotional isolation. There is no plot device which is not used, no chain un-yanked or string un-pulled. The plot of the temptation story is powerful because we can see ourselves within the story. We can feel the sun on our neck. We begin to share with Jesus the emptiness of belly and soul and we begin to hallucinate from mal-nourishment and isolation. We've all been alone like this before.

We've all been Spirit-compelled, and hungry for meaning in an unrelenting wasteland. All of us will go to that lonely wilderness. For the last year all of us have been in that wilderness, seemingly left alone. What will you discover, who will you become when you confront the adder in the arid wilderness?

A DISTURBING DEVELOPMENT

As you may know, we are not yet to the "bad" part of this tale. The most disturbing part of this whole story is, that just when Jesus is coming to grips with loneliness, just as He is starting to notice the same familiar animals creeping around Him, just as he sees the same lingering mirages of food, shelter, and solace he realizes that He is not really alone.

The dragon followed Him. The snake slithered from garden, to city, to wasteland. Just when we, like Jesus come to think that we have grown comfortable with the most unforgiving of environments just when we are finding a way to first survive and thrive then the serpents hiss, the dragon's croak echoes in our fevered brain. "It does not have to be this way." "Jesus, Jesus, *Jesus*: I have the answer!" "I can fill your belly. I can give you the world. I can deliver from all this discomfort." The same old, unchanging, ancient temptations, repackaged, repainted, regurgitated.

The desert can bring out the best in human character. Survival requires discipline of mind, spirit, and body. Life in a harsh environment requires individuals to discipline their desires, balancing want and need. Humans will always need desert defined discipline in times of temptation. It must be cultivated. It must be developed. We must go to the desert to test our strength, to hone the muscles of faith. We must go willingly so that we might achieve the maturity which will allow us to overcome temptation without bowing to other idolatrous threats like pride and selfishness.

Like Jesus we need to go to the desert and find there not a permanent dwelling place but a place of preparation. A place of refinement. A place where we can be tempered for the work that God intends for us.

And it is here that our adversary disturbs our peace. First, he attacks our strengths then he makes a move against our weaknesses. He questions motives and knowingly winks at our assertions of fidelity. He's been alone with "us" before. Adam, and Abram, and David, and Solomon. He knows that the key is using human appetite. Use a hunger for food to create a hunger for recognition. A thirsty man thinks not only of his parched throat but also of the way that power satisfies other inner cravings. Attacking God will only make a faithful man more resolute. Don't denigrate God, (at least not yet), elevate the individual instead. Don't remove God from His pedestal, widen it, and include this brave individual, this daring soul out here in the wild. "Why are you here Jesus? So brave! So resolute! Such courage, such a divine response!" Soon the weak minded, soporifically stumbling amidst the wasted vegetation begins to see that here in the desert they *can* be the hero of the story. And that is when the snake, the adversary must be recognized for what and who he is.

Antagonist

Satan. The Devil. The Accuser. It seems only fitting that a character who first appears in Biblical story polluting the purity of Eden should be seen, at the outset of Jesus' ministry, here in a desolate wasteland. It's almost as if he's saying "look what we've done to the place! Me, human Empire, civilization, the pleasures of the flesh combined with the corruption of all forms of corporation. Bam! Here it is! Paradise is not only lost it's become a blasted wasteland. Yay me!"

Unlike God, Satan does not have unlimited power. Like us, he is fallen. Of sketchy angelic background, Satan, at some point decided that submission was not his style and that he would rather roam and ruin earth than serve the Creator God. So, from jabbing at Job to jabbering in Jonah's ear, in one way or another, he tries to divert the faithful from their task to honor God and to live righteously.

Some are easy. Sex. Power. Riches. Those who can be seduced by the pleasures of the flesh, the desire of the eyes and vital power of pride[3] are easily distracted. Once their attention is turned away from God and focused on self it is just a matter of time until faithful resolve melts. All this loneliness, all this desert space is the perfect environment to create envy and resentment. "Shouldn't others prepare as well? Where is everyone else?" (Pride is introduced.) "I do not deserve to be treated this way!" ("Oh, is that envy I see?") When the faithful is isolated, and cast out into the desert the loudest voice in the chorus of doubt is the mocking of the adversary.

When the eyes sting with sweat and the brow is burnt by the sun, when the mind is clouded by exhaustion and prayerful anxiety, it is then that the ancient antagonist attacks. It is when days have passed and weariness has grown, that Satan requisitions all his manifold methods-everything he has crafted to destroy mankind since that far away morning in paradise and prepares to undermine the Son of God with the simplest of suggestions.

It is in this sort of a triumphant spirit that the Accuser of the brethren sidles up to the Son of Man and makes his pitch. "Would you like a sandwich? Ham, perhaps? (Snicker, snicker . . . just kidding.) Corned beef? How about a nice, cold drink of spring water?" The real issue is not ever, not really, the immediate discomforts of the flesh, do not become confused. The actual issue is not the limits of flesh and blood. The heart of the battle, the issue most fully in play is the ultimate assertion of allegiance.

Allegiance

That's what the Devil is interested in. Hunger, thirst, and isolation are means to an end. Real temptation not only aims for the dethroning or marginalizing of God through disobedience, but it also seeks to elevate the creature and put him in charge. Now, Satan knows that Jesus is different, that He is not only fully human but that He also is fully Divine. All the better! If Jesus can be

3. 1 John 2.16

27

"turned" then his grand scheme to destroy and despoil creation can continue. If Jesus Himself is unable to bear full allegiance while blasted by the desert sun, then no one possibly can!

His goal then, his true end, is to get us to worship self. So, he works to feed that hunger, diminish that thirst, sever that singular bond with our creator. When we are distracted by our needs, when our needs become wants, when our wants are transformed and intensified into destructive desires—it is then that basic human instinct morphs into temptation. It is then that we forget our first and highest allegiance and neglect our responsibility to answer to God. All because the slight whisper of want has become the ranting, untamable beast of need. In succumbing to this process, we chase the unobtainable goal of "being like God." Maybe you've heard that one before? Not realizing that in pursuing the path of self-aggrandizing personal deification, in bowing our knee to the unquenchable craving of self we are ultimately bowing down to the Dragon. The same dragon who once upon a time promised the same exact thing for the low, low price of a single bite of forbidden fruit.

Even in the heat of desert isolation we must come to understand that like our primordial parents awaiting God's daily walk in the garden the choice is always ours. Satan's cunning voice will always be there. He will always show up at the worst possible moment offering whatever tempts our current weakness. The bread he offers can both sustain our strength and sap our determination to grow increasingly faithful. He offers a fame which is fleeting, a peace which is pretend, and an empire of empty promises. All he has to give is a corrupted copy of the human community that God establishes on the word and work of Jesus. The Church is built on selfless love. Hell is built on love of self.

Jesus has come into this high desert place for this very moment. To see all the corrupt and blasted work of sinful man juxtaposed with the possibility of Kingdom. The gnawing for food must be realized in a passion for service. Thirst must motivate mercy. Lonely prayer in the wilderness will provide the foundation for private prayer in times of crowded days of ministry and equally lonely nights of waiting and watching. The question Jesus is dealing with, the question we all must deal with, will I be faithful, focused, and loyal?

Everything is a loyalty test. Everything is a pledge or denial of allegiance. Every choice we choose, every voice to which we give ear each and all of them is asking us, "Who is in charge?" In the wilderness all the distractions, deflections and redefinitions of the central question are stripped away. What our bodies feel, and our minds ponder is not so much the pain as the purpose. One cannot really hear when civilization is rioting in our ears. We cannot think when our minds are clouded with the normal verities of our daily experience. We cannot focus on God when those dear to us call for our undivided attention. We cannot really understand what God is asking until we are alone with Him in circumstances where we can isolate His voice from all those other competing voices and know completely and distinctly what loyalty requires.

Satan will shout. He will provide other outlets upon which we can settle our silent assent. Hunger and thirst point to self. Fame, glory, fortune, and Empire point beyond imagination not only to comfort and relief but also to some presumed sense of vindication. Yet what he offers diminishes when compared with what he demands in return. He too wants loyalty. What seems to elevate self, escorts him into the throne room of one's heart.

Everything is a loyalty test. It only seems as if temptation is about what happens to us or what we choose or how we react. Maybe that is why the Father does not feature in this desert temptation story. Jesus was surely praying during His time of fasting. The Father's voice was heard when He was baptized. The Spirit had compelled His desert retreat. Yet the Father leaves the Son in the desert alone with the elements, alone with the physical torments, alone with the tempter. For in those circumstances, the pledge of allegiance each must offer the Father—even when it is Jesus who is so asked—may not be compelled.

Think of the opportunities you have had in a wilderness year, a desert year, an isolated year. How have you fared when hunger and thirst and human fortune seemed to be at issue? Did isolation increase or reduce the space between you and God? Each of us inhabited our own slice of this isolated, socially distanced reality. Was it a time of conflict for you or a time of contentment? Each day of our lives is filled with opportunity as well as challenges. Were you more focused on what was excluded from your time in the wilderness or did you focus on what you retained? Your wits? Your capacity to relate to God individually? Did you read your Bible more? Perhaps you learned something new and different about prayer. Did you discover a new author, listen to a new composer, or cultivate a new skill? What did you do in the desert? What did you do with this tempering, potentially life-changing gift? Were there times of celebration or was it one long, complaint-filled, self-centered, pitiful slog?

Did you realize that Satan was peeking through your window challenging your loyalty by attacking your flesh and planting doubts in your alienated psyche? Of course not! That's not how we think of it. We have ways of circling the wagons and defending ourselves against the ordinary and the obvious. History teaches us that desperate and difficult times are the desert experiences that can strengthen our resolve, calibrate our loyalty, and deepen our allegiance in order that we can be prepared for future acts of service. We understand that—until it happens. Then, in that moment of deprivation where God can finally get our attention and the scheming of the Adversary can be exposed for what it really is, at that critical juncture we look desert temptation in the eye, and blink. Rather than undergoing refinement we react with resentment. Rather than using isolation to drive us deeper into the Word of God we are driven deeper into a culture of complaint. Rather than waiting on God's Spirit; we whine.

In 2020 A.D. as well as 30 A.D. —everything is a loyalty test. Jesus shows us how to express that loyalty in the very throes of desperate, discouraging, deserted circumstances. We are not always paying attention.

RESPONSIBLE RESOLUTION

Personal integrity is rejecting stolen food when you are starving. Consistent faithfulness means obedience even when it seems as if you have been abandoned. Resolution requires us to turn our back on false messiahs who promise a palace they have no right to offer in exchange for a fealty they have no right to ask. If someone ever asks you what Jesus' temptation in the wilderness means, read the preceding summary to them.

Of course, the time we spent social distancing in Twenty-Twenty was different than Jesus' time in the wilderness. Except for the temptation part. And ours was a technologically enabled shared experience, thanks to Zoom, FaceTime, social media, and text-messaging.

Though Jesus undertook His desert separation deliberately and purposefully He discovered dimensions of faith which would not have been possible in the comforts of Nazareth or through the Sabbath-by-Sabbath Synagogue readings and prayers which had been central in His spiritual development. Unlike everyone else in the crowd around John, He heard a different message, a message which resonated with His own growing Messianic consciousness and emerging life vision. In a world filled with much deprivation and depravity He knew that Kingdom would have difficulty having an impact on the masses of humanity, desperately looking for answers in such dire times. In wilderness isolation, Jesus prepared Himself for the intense immersion in crowds, congregations, masses, mobs, and riots which would typify His public ministry. The things He would do and speak would evoke tremendous emotions and generate enormous crowds. How appealing! How alluring! How addictive! Attractive!

And so, Spirit-compelled, Jesus puts as much distance as possible between the beckoning crowds and Himself. Time to gather His thoughts. Time to evaluate the plan. Time to organize His program of teaching. Time to consider what kind of men He would need. Clearly, many of His disciples were already known to Him. Some were perhaps even related to Him. Regardless of where they came from, He would use His own wilderness interlude to contemplate the future. He would consider how to train emerging leaders. He would contemplate how to cast a new vision for Kingdom-shaped living in a world dominated by Empire.

Do not think that Jesus was idle in the wilderness. He did not just sit there counting lizards and trying to forget His own hunger. The synoptics make it quite clear; He stormed out of the wilderness into the Galilee preaching and teaching, calling, and cajoling, healing, and helping. Jesus left the wilderness with a plan. He formed that plan while there in the wilderness. Beyond temptation the desert provided a place and a time of intense preparation a final prelude to a three-year assault by the Son of God upon the kingdom of darkness. Of course, the snake himself would slither into the desert to disrupt and distract Jesus' purposeful retreat there. So, in parallel Jesus must remain true to the controlling purpose which drove Him to the desert and respond to the very real temptations offered Him by the old, familiar desert dragon.

The reality of the temptations that Jesus experienced, and of which we read is conditioned by both their immediacy and their consequence. Humanity's garden nemesis offered to Jesus the same ill-gotten gain offered Adam. Know now. Have now. Be satisfied now. Compromise a little, to gain a lot. Just a small nibble of bread, a slight bend of the knee, a spectacular feat of super-human ability. Satan's bargain always seems to be: "give a little to gain the world!" Jesus' response: "Our lives are entirely in God's hands." Our daily bread, our daily worship, our daily safety. We are creatures made to be both independent and dependent at the same time. In the wilderness, wholly alone, we along with Jesus, can be reminded of the great strengths with which we are created along with the great weaknesses. The strong of mind know that when the body and will are weakened our reliance upon God's own faithfulness, so clearly revealed to us in the Bible, is essential for our survival. The snake is tricky. Yet his chicanery reveals his most basic limitation. He is a copycat. He is a killer. He is a deceiver. He is sly, and salacious, and desperate. But he did not create this world he so desperately wants to destroy. And we, the creatures at its center, for whom his hate burns the brightest are capable of reading and retaining our creators' thoughts after Him. Thus, fortified we are able, following in the footsteps of Jesus, to say "no" when the serpent substitutes allurement for accusation.

It is far too tempting (do excuse the pun) to respond to the tempter with anger and accusation, reflecting his approach to us. It always feels good to respond in kind to those who would seek to destroy us. Hitting back is practically reflexive. In doing so, we unwittingly accomplish ourselves what various temptations could never do. We reflect whom we follow. If we really wish to reflect the life of Jesus in our own it will require that we consider what He did in the wilderness. We may not be confronted with the same temptations. We will confront the same adversary. The responsible resolution Jesus sought to the attacks of His antagonist did not involve responding in kind. He did not argue. He did not hit back. He did not return insult for insult. He did not defend Himself or the appetites He denied. He did not focus on Himself when isolation offered Him that pathway to celebrating self. It may be difficult for us to think of it this way, but I doubt if Jesus raised His voice, became agitated or emotional in any way. He simply seems to conduct Himself with great self-confidence in a potentially destructive conversation with His greatest adversary. How can He be so cool, calm, and collected in the searing desert heat? Satan thought the circumstances, he thought the environment would prove decisive. Alone, yet not alienated. Hungry, but not desperate. Ambitious for Kingdom, not Imperial glory. Jesus only looked vulnerable to Satan and those who shared his fallen outlook. He was the expert in losing paradise and reducing Eden to ashes. Jesus was and is the expert in speaking into the Abyss to create order, structure, and beauty out of nothingness. Satan fell prey to his own temptation! He should have stayed far, far away from the desert. He was no match and never had been, for the Creative-World-Making Word of God.

Jesus models for every socially distanced, relationship-famished believer what a relationship with God can do for our mind, body, and spirit. We need not see our current struggle as bondage.

The desert is only desolate for those who cannot see beyond the sand and tortured vegetation. The wilderness is only wasteland for those who cannot see within it the retrievable vestiges of the paradise we once lost.

Jesus responded to that lying snake not by outshouting the liar but by quoting and applying the relevant words of scripture in a timely fashion and on point. It was not Sunday School. It was not theoretical. It was not showing off so that the local Rabbi would pick you for his side when it was Torah quiz time. Nope. Jesus responded to lies with the truth of scripture. He not only knew it, and quoted it: He lived it.

2

Garden Prayer

In a Garden Paradise
Adam and Eve (we as well)
Enjoyed the morning fellowship
Until the bite and then they fell.
Since that moment long ago
Another garden waits.
where second Adam prepares and prays
For Satan's violent blow.
Paradise Renewed requires
The Faithful Son to give
His life for yours and mine
That with Him we might live.

A FAMILIAR STORY

How is it that Jesus found Himself *alone* in the Garden? The week had largely been busy. A crowd hailed Him, cheered Him, sang, and danced for Him as He entered Jerusalem. For most of His ministry there had been crowds. Sometimes just groups milling about hoping to catch a snatch of the wisdom for which He was becoming famous. There were a few occasions when the crowd was well-ordered and seemed intent on learning and applying what He had to say. On those occasions He was able to be more systematic. On those days He was able to pull together some of His favorite metaphors, combine them with His creative reimagining of the Hebrew Bible and begin the process of casting His new Kingdom vision.

There were a few times it got downright scary. Once in His hometown after synagogue service, first the learned leaders, then the few wealthy in Nazareth, finally the full congregation became a ranting, rioting, railing mob. They drove Him to the edge of town with murderous intent, yet He was able to slip away and make good His escape.

That was His first mob. Not the last. On another occasion, filled with bread and pickled fish that He had compassionately provided after a long day's wilderness teaching, the crowd, becoming restless, began to chant His name. They were dancing and singing. Now shouting, crying out really, proclaiming His name they skated close to the edge of the border between Kingdom and Empire. "Make Him King! Force Him if we must!" They had glimpsed a vision of His abilities and mistakenly believed that He and His miraculous powers could be harnessed to national ambitions for power, majesty, expansion, aggrandizement. They had hoped that He could front, fund, and feed their own attempt at Empire. He demurred, drifted out of the crowd unnoticed and probably reflected prayerfully upon all the bad things that happened when groups become crowds and crowds became mobs.

Jerusalem was somewhat different. He had been here before and like all Jewish men participated in the temple rituals. He had brought sacrifices. He had been through the ritual baths. He understood the power of symbol, and the overwhelming grandeur of a building dedicated to the worship of the Creator God, whom He called Father-and whose city, and house He and all Israel was entering. The city was always full. During feasts, and festivals, and pilgrimage it expanded like a skin swelling with the released spirits of fermenting wine (likely metaphor there). More and more people. More needs. More desperation. Deeper poverty. More intense fervor.

Because the city was so volatile during festal seasons the Romans took extra precautions to insure a "peaceful" celebration. For them peaceful meant profitable. Whatever the natives wanted to do and in whoever's divine name they wanted to do it was fine with the Emperor and his extended governing apparatus. Basically, everything was allowed. And taxed. So, yes nearly anything was permitted so long as it was profitable.

The journey had been the same as always. The same route through the same villages, across the same miles. It had been somewhat more active. It seemed that every town, every village, every caravan-crossed oasis between the Galilee and Judea became a venue. A place to speak a place, to heal. Sometimes just a place to frolic with a few children and spend a few moments in more intense, focused instruction with His disciples. Jericho, Bethany, the descent from the Mount of Olives, the final climb into the city.

Recalling the ancient words of sacred song He had made arrangements to enter the city in a manner fit for a King; a Messiah. The foundation had been adequately laid. His disciples were far from perfect but up to the task before them. In the future, with the addition of an ever-present advocate, they would carry on His vision and proclaim the coming Kingdom. This would come after His own final glorification and ascent. Now for the first time during His earthly sojourn, it was time to be publicly proclaimed King. No more secrets. No more hints. He is finished laying the ground-work. It is time to be announced as the cornerstone. This will be the first time and the only time.

So, He donkeyed up and entered in triumph the City of the great King. He, Himself (the I AM) being that king.

Some of the Crowd became so enthused that they ripped off their outer garments and flung them into the roadway in an act of submission. Others took palm branches and alternatively waved and flung them in similar token of worship and affection. More and more joined in! The celebration grew! The roar of the crowds

rose the swelling melodious singing of Israel's ancient Songs of
Ascent!

> "And the crowds that went before him and that followed
> him were shouting, "Hosanna to the Son of David!
> Blessed is he who comes in the name of the Lord! Ho-
> sanna in the highest!"" (Matthew 21:9 ESV)

Under watchful Roman eyes the temple authorities began to
grow concerned about this popular prophet who multiplied bread
as if it were the manna of ancient miracle, and who created crowds
out of a few pre-occupied peasants from the marketplace.

The hustle and bustle the hurrying and preparing and gathering and teaching and moving from place to place had gone on for
weeks and had culminated in this celebratory parade in the City
of David.

And it really didn't slow down after that. Next, He went to
the Temple and found it still a rather disappointing place. It was
not, of course, His first visit to this, the historical and geographi-
cal heart of the Jewish world. For many Jews, familiarity with the
Temple had created a sort of holy contempt, not for what it was
intended to be, not for what it represented, not for all the theological truth it symbolized. It disappointed because culture, commerce
and Empire had encroached upon it. The temple had become a
center of culture, of banking, of social cohesion. Worship occurred
yet it was no longer what drove the events in and around the sacred precincts. The purpose of prayer and the wonder of worship
were eclipsed by more prosaic, more human activities. And so,
Jesus experienced a rising anger. The purpose of the Temple was
neglected. The holiness of the Temple compromised. His righteous
indignation rose for the contempt He saw. A contempt borne of
sophisticated and long-standing misuse of a central theological
motif of Hebrew religion. Rather than serving as a place of prayer,
and worship, and devotion it was performing the common social
function of market, bank, and cultural symbol. Markets were
important. Banking, despite constant complaints throughout history, performs an important social function. And every significant

society ever has had deeply entrenched and meaningful cultural symbols. Yet Jesus knew that for all its functional significance the Temple was failing as a place where people found meaning. The temple was losing its primary role of being the place where people could come to experience God's presence. It was for that very reason that scribes and pharisees were supplanting priests and levites as spiritual leaders in the minds of the people. Things were so bad that the Essenes who were descendants of priests themselves had moved out into the desert to protest everything that the Temple had become.

While Jesus had garnered for Himself the reputation of one who would not go along to get along, He had not, to this point in His public ministry, played the role of provocateur. He had hinted that the spiritual leaders of the people had become power-hungry and fortune conscious. He had alluded to the fact that the Law was being taught in such a way that it was robbed of its transformative power. After all, though it did serve as the foundation for both the "secular" and religious law throughout Israel's history and now in the era of formative Judaism; clearly the secular function rose out of and was endemically related to the spiritual purpose for which it had been first intended. In fact, much of what Jesus said and did was intended to replace the formal, repetitive, merely functional adherence to rules with a transformative experience of what He Himself mediated through His presence: The Kingdom of God.

And so, job one on this Passover would be to try and, at least symbolically if not more permanently, at least, not yet, restore a proper sense of decorum, decency, and duty to the sacred space. Kick out the thieves, release the animals (yet another small irony there) and announce the Father's displeasure. Jesus knew that this Passover week would be different because He knew how it would end.

So, from that incident things grew. Constant questioning from the clever, the conniving, and the confused. Exegesis of Torah. Answers to trivia and some looking for tidbits of inside information which would help them to make sense of an increasingly senseless world.

When times get intense the confused and timid look for an authority figure to tell them everything will be just fine. Accordingly, many members of the crowd were merely looking to be reassured. They trusted their teachers; Scribe, Pharisee, Sadducee, the spare Essene who may have been hanging about. The common people trusted the learned and literate to ask the right questions of Jesus and to formulate a proper understanding of who He was, what He intended, and how He planned to supplant the malicious machine of Empire with the empathetic entity called Kingdom.

And the cultured elite failed. The professional and professorial classes failed. The leaders of the people, the ones they trusted they all failed. Rather than being filled with curiosity they were filled with contempt. Instead of a thirst for knowledge they approached Jesus awash in dreams of their own erudition. They could have come to Him for insight. Instead, driven by vanity, pride, and a lust for power they turned what could have been a quest for transformative knowledge into a petty fight over the most piddling and pedantic minutia available for debate. They wished to prove themselves to Jesus and elevate themselves in the minds of the populace. The people were confused and Jesus, unimpressed. He even told one story where He emphatically concluded "the vineyard will be taken away and given to other tenants." Everyone knew that He was accusing the leaders of the people of failing to lead, ignoring the truth, mishandling the scriptures, and undermining the faith of the common people. Jesus, having spent the week in every conceivable forum for debate began to focus on the final steps to be taken.

So, toward the middle of the week Jesus began to turn his attention away from the crowds and to consider His last days, the final moments of intimate instruction with his closest companions. He had for weeks been teaching them about the final journey and its ultimate outcome. One moment they seemed to understand the next they were perplexed, combative, and sullen. The passing of time allows us the luxury of judging the disciples through the harsh lens of hindsight. Surely if you or I were there we would remain focused during the long week of instruction, debate, ministry, and celebration. Whatever Jesus was planning, despite the opposition and hardships we would expect that our time with Jesus, our personal experiences with Him, had hardened us—as surely it hardened them against all forms of doubt or skepticism. Jesus had taught them well. When we read in the New Testament of all that He did to open the eyes and minds and perspective of His disciples we are rightly awed by the foundation which he laid in their lives and by the very model of patient discipleship which He provides. To this day when other more modern terms are available, we describe the process of coming to faith, maturing, learning, apprenticing, engaging in mission—all of this we call discipleship.

Jesus knew the journey was ending. Though they may have suspected that there was a change in the air they certainly did not think of it in the stark, drastic terms Jesus had been using during the long weeks of their journey toward Jerusalem. Maybe they missed it because they had become so attuned to His aphorisms, focused on His wordplays, and fixated on His metaphors that they had forgotten that metaphors have referents. His images pointed to realities which were about to become present. They overlooked the fact that His aphorisms spoke Kingdom judgement against the pretense of all forms of Empire. Wordplays and puns came with punchlines and those who were the "butt" of the joke often resented what was insinuated.

As phase one of Kingdom ministry wound down Jesus had a few formative moments left to spend with those to whom He was entrusting His legacy. Much of what we do in worship, the central acts, and facts at the heart of Christian observance were established in the collective memory of the Church during that final 60 hours which Jesus spent in Jerusalem. Pouring His mind into His teaching. Pouring His heart into His disciples. Pouring His life out for many. So, as the Passover approached, after a furious week of diverse ministry activities Jesus set aside an evening to be with His embryonic Church before they set out on their first truly adverse, formative adventure.

Passion week with Him would prepare the Church for Kingdom ministry in His absence. Soon they would learn to rely upon the promised Holy Spirit, the text of the Hebrew Bible which had formed them all, and Jesus' own words of Kingdom-organizing revelation. For this final evening He was there with them in loving, serving fellowship.

Before the storm? Rest. Relaxation. Celebration. The highlight of their Year and one of the central focal points of their national and religious history. A time of reflection, rejoicing and reconsideration of God's work among mankind.

One more party. One more highlight. Would they remember things he had told them like:

> 34 And Jesus said to them, "Can you make wedding guests fast while the bridegroom is with them? 35 The days will come when the bridegroom is taken away from them, and then they will fast in those days."[1]

Yes, the time for fasting would soon come. He knew that they would pass a fretful, hungry, sleepless weekend. But first the feast. First the party. A final moment of joy before the breaking wave of the stored-up sin of all humanity would fall upon Him and break his body.

He sent some of the lads to make proper arrangements. A large enough room. A large enough lamb. Enough bread and wine. This would be a final gathering with those who had left their livelihoods, left their families, left the familiar lake, left the Galilee to follow him on this journey. We do not know whether or not Jesus had gathered His intimate disciples with Him before to celebrate Passover. We assume that He did. Yet the Gospels are not tabloids, there were no paparazzi to catch Him or those around Him on their last round of shopping before the big night. As faithful and observant Jews Passover was without a doubt a perennial and central concern. Yet clearly Jesus had orchestrated events in order that this particular Passover would not only provide the signature highlight for one of the founding moments of the Church but would come to be understood as the very last Passover of its kind. After that night, after those words, Passover was forever changed

---

1. Luke 5:34–35 (ESV)

both for formative Judaism and for earliest Christianity. These sibling faiths would forever look to that one night for answers to what unified and separated them. Whichever one chooses and however one behaves the clear differentiating factor in all Passovers before that night and all Passovers after, was Jesus. He infused what had been a people defining, even segregating feast and made it a unifying point for all fallen humanity. He gathered us not merely around the good things of the earth, bread, and wine and lamb. He took those simple elements and used them to symbolize His saving relationship to His fallen creation. The disciples may have thought they were celebrating one more Passover as they did year upon year. After this night. After this week. After this—everything would be different.

They celebrated the feast. Like all men everywhere on these sorts of occasions there was laughter. There was joy. They told the story of Exodus. They remembered the heroes of old. They likely speculated about their own little story—which seemed so small compared to the feats of Moses and Joshua and David. Would they be remembered? And what for? They were jealous about the reputation of Jesus. They had spent a lifetime listening and learning from Rabbis of all stripes and schools. From the moment they had heard Jesus teach they knew that what He said was different from all the others. Jesus spoke with an authority which was personal. It was not derivative or secondary. He spoke with an instinctive, primary understanding of what people needed, why they sinned and what could be done about it. When Jesus spoke, there was immediacy. When Jesus taught it was an act of new creation. When Jesus spoke, He spoke like God.

The men conversed. Every large group has a pecking order, and this band of brothers, this cohort of disciples was no different. There were flesh and blood brothers in the group. As family does, they surely recalled when this uncle or that one over-cooked the lamb or spilled wine on grandma's special tablecloth. There were colleagues—business partners. Men who share commerce together naturally congregate and share the collective lore of the trade. There was small talk. Those who cooked and prepared carried on the typical conversations of those sharing an important task. Maybe they sang. Though the text is silent on the issue it is highly likely that there were women present. Later, when what was basically the same group gathered on Pentecost there were 120 gathered in what was presumably the same room. So even if the broader traveling group of disciples was not there for the Passover feast there may have been a few women; in fact they were likely the ones chatting as they roasted, and baked, and poured, and prepared. In virtually every human gathering there is someone who brings his discontent with him. For one reason or another there are some people who will never be entirely happy. Never quite enough money for supplies. Resources wasted which could have been used to feed the poor. Opportunities squandered to beat back the darkness of Empire. Judas whisperingly muttered to himself, unaware that Jesus was aware.

He knew-as he always knew-that someone had been tempted, someone had been bribed, one had been turned. Then, there were words between them. Harsh and offending words. Uncomfortable questions were asked. Tensions rose as bold assertions flew behind cautious gazes. He knew that the others would be shocked and offended. He was not. He gave the nod, dipped the morsel, and bid Judas to quickly go and do what had been decided. Then he had one more new, additional feature to add to the feast; something not intended to merely secure the foundational memory of the past but to be a continual reminder of what all of his work was intended to accomplish and to point to its ultimate resolution, envisioning a moment when all creation would be cleansed of its sinfulness and Kingdom would come in nuptial celebration. Till then a morsel of bread and a communal sip of wine would need to be enough to remind His people that this sacrificial and sacerdotal mission, upon which only He could embark, would indeed make all things new. They would sing a hymn to remind them of a new song, a kingdom song and then went to a garden; a little reminder of the paradise once lost that His work would regain.

A DISTURBING DEVELOPMENT

Every one of them, every disciple, slept. It was all but inevitable. The whole entourage was tired. It had been a long and exhausting week on top of a long and exhausting journey filled with ministry and mystery, storms stilled, and stories told. They had walked the breadth of the region. They witnessed and participated in incredible demonstrations of the power of God. Jesus was filled with strength and purpose, and they certainly drew upon His reserves. Jesus provided the example, the energy, and the enthusiasm they needed for the work to which He had called them. The work for which He had prepared them.

But as for now, they were tired. Passover was a time of feasting and reflection. Having left their families, villages, fishing, farming and all other kinds of business endeavors they feasted and celebrated with this new and empowering group centered around Jesus. But feasting was feasting and after such a journey, weeks and months of emotion, and a filling meal they were already nodding off as they sang their song and headed out into the evening.

Even as they relaxed after the meal the natural pecking order reemerged. Proximity. Age. Perspective. We don't know why some were in the inner circle and why others were not. It is an accident of history which was not recorded in any of the Gospels. It stands to reason, as is always the case in virtually any group, that besides the innermost circle around Jesus there were other small groupings of disciples. Men who were far away from home and who grouped together because of a shared vocation or shared family members, or shared perspectives. Maybe some of them were just more gregarious and others tended to be loners. And now, one was missing. We don't know whether the disciples really missed Judas until he reappears at the critical moment. If they thought he was performing some significant task then there was little reason to suspect him of any malfeasance. They had shared a pleasant meal together and now, moving to the mountain garden in self-selecting groups they intended to enjoy the rest of the evening together.

Maybe some were asleep on their feet as they walked together upon the twisting mountain pass. Maybe they were joking and joshing the way young men on the march have always done. Surely, they laughed an occasional, quiet, respectful laugh in the growing darkness.

Having arrived at the garden, still grouped in twos or threes, they settled down. Matthew's full account of the story reads like this.

> 36 *Then Jesus went with them to a place called Gethsemane, and he said to his disciples, "Sit here, while I go over there and pray." 37 And taking with him Peter and the two sons of Zebedee, he began to be sorrowful and troubled. 38 Then he said to them, "My soul is very sorrowful, even to death; remain here, and watch with me." 39 And going a little farther he fell on his face and prayed, saying, "My Father, if it be possible, let this cup pass from me; nevertheless, not as I will, but as you will." 40 And he came to the disciples and found them sleeping. And he said to Peter, "So, could you not watch with me one hour? 41 Watch and pray that you may not enter into temptation. The spirit indeed is willing, but the flesh is weak." 42 Again, for the second time, he went away and prayed, "My Father, if this cannot pass unless I drink it, your will be done." 43 And again he came and found them sleeping, for their eyes were heavy. 44 So, leaving them again, he went away and prayed for the third time, saying the same words again. 45 Then he came to the disciples and said to them, "Sleep and take your rest later on. See, the hour is at hand, and the Son of Man is betrayed into the hands of sinners. 46 Rise, let us be going; see, my betrayer is at hand. "Matthew 26:36–46 (ESV)*

For the faithful Christian these words bear something of a challenge. Surely *I* would not be so slothful and egregiously thankless as to sleep as the Master prayed? Not me. Never. Jesus surely heard that a lot from His disciple-companions. They were only growing into a ministry for which He had been preparing Himself for all eternity. Yet, after months of following, hearing, and participating He had reason to think that some of them could at least spend the night with Him in watchful prayer.

Jesus appears disappointed. Not for the silence. He more than made up for the silence with His own prayer. It was not the loneliness because he was really never alone. His communion with the Father was so complete, so enriching that He did not feel any separation at all, even here on the cusp of the cross. And it was not the recalcitrance of the disciples. He was used to that. Much of His methodology as a teacher was about breaking down their defenses, getting beyond their natural skepticism, burrowing beneath their bullheadedness.

He was disappointed because He knew what was coming and how unprepared they really were. He relished the opportunity to watch and pray with them, but they needed Him far more than He needed them. If they only knew. Whether because of fatigue, full bellies, or the wine, they were missing the last night on earth with Him.

What have you made of the Gethsemane moments in your life? Have you staggered up narrow mountain passes in the company of the Savior only to let go of His hand in your darkest moment? Oh, I'm sorry, perhaps that is too personal. Yet, we need such challenges. Twenty-twenty has been a long slog of a year for all of us. We have all travelled through hard, lonely places and dark, despairing times. We have felt as though we were isolated in a desert. Or keeping watch while our companions sleep through the nightmare. Many are aimless. Many lack purpose. Not a few have abandoned all hope. But there are some among us who, rather than creasing Hs forehead with disappointment, have brought genuine joy to Jesus. They have sought Him in those desert places. They have been awake and alert to what the Spirit teaches in the whispers of the solemn watches of the night when snippets of memorized scripture animate their dreams. These alert disciples have spent their time, not in aimless wandering but in disciplined and deliberate devotion. Some have sought His face, listened for His voice and learned how to respond to the solitude as He did.

Some have aligned their purposes more fully with His and have grown more hopeful even as those around us have been in despair.

Maybe the sequestration journey is over. Perhaps the pandemic is passing us by like the avenging Angel passing over our worried culture as it once passed over Egypt. Maybe it will come and go and provide new challenges in the future. Like those disciples we look around and find the faithful, remember the fallen, reprimand the fickle. There is such opportunity. To feast with the Master. To hear His voice. To pray in his presence. To embrace Him in our solitude. We have too much to gain to go to sleep now. Will you weaken so much that, here at the end of the test, your flesh grows numb, your eyes grow heavy, and sleep comes unbidden?

RESPONSIBLE RESOLUTION

How did Jesus deal with the loneliness and isolation He felt in the looming shadow of the Cross? He resolved these impending issues by continuing in a faithful engagement with the Father. He did not understand His situation as one of loneliness and isolation. He was wearied from the journey and perhaps worn from the constant pressures of ministry, but He never felt like he was estranged from the Father.

His disciples were worn down with fatigue. They finally realized the enormity of the hour. The cross was now a real and looming threat. Their faith was being challenged in a new and personal way. They were loyal to Jesus but the spiraling of difficult circumstances obscured the nearness of the Father. All seemed lost to them. Rather than feeling God's presence in solitude, they imagined His absence. They were now faced with perhaps the final opportunity for shared prayer and it eluded them. They just couldn't keep their eyes open.

Were they being short-sighted and irresponsible? Perhaps. Was their faith wavering? It would seem so. Jesus had poured his life into their instruction but on a darkening evening in even darker times it was hard to stay awake. We easily criticize their failing from the safety of thousands of miles and thousands of years.

Though the disciples were the church in embryonic form to put it bluntly, we were not there, we don't really know, and we should stop pretending in our far-removed courageous pride that we do. How many of us have slept, or are continuing to sleep through our generation's Gethsemene moment?

In dealing with their "failure" Jesus responds with kindness and words of support. He continued to serve them even as his own time was drawing short. He never stopped leading, He never stopped being who He was.

Beyond His loving attention to His disciples Jesus never lost the broader vision and mission which brought Him to that hill-top garden in the first place. The whole reason for Immanuel being *there*-the purpose for Him being here amongst us was to drink the cup prepared from before the foundation of the world. He understood that if he were to falter now, if He were to back away from or shirk the painful responsibility of betrayal and cross then not only would His earthly ministry have been in vain but the entire plan of salvation-indeed, the entire scope of Salvation-history would have been for naught.

Steadfast in submission yet boldly assertive in prayer He approaches the Father not with an attitude borne of His equality in Deity but with a humility accepted for its utility. The Word who had been made flesh, who had walked the forsaken, fallen creation, communes with the Father in whom, through whom, and by whose strength the coming ordeal was to be endured and ultimately overcome. Jesus prayed not as a condemned man going to His death but as a victorious Lord who understood that the road to victory would wind perilously and painfully through the valley of the shadow of death. "Your will-not mine". "In your strength-not mine." God's age-long, passionate pursuit of wayward humanity ending first in the terminal breath-whisper of death then echoing with the triumphant shout of resurrection.

The only resolution to His garden-loneliness was surrender. Victory would come not in seeking a way around the coming storm of the cross but in seeking the Father's strength so that He might go through this empowering passion which could only then become the means of releasing the fallen from the grip of death and restoring creation to its destiny.

In looking at Jesus in the Garden we find a model for how each of us should face the garden interludes of our own lives. They come in many fashions. Perhaps someone you love died prematurely. Maybe you have suffered a broken heart. For some Christians the peril is nearly as real as was Jesus'. Betrayal. Loneliness. Beating. Humiliation. Yes, even death. How you and I face Gethsemane largely determines how well we have understood the cross and the empowering victory of the empty tomb. When we assume that the Christian life is painless, we do not value what Jesus achieved for us nor do we understand why it had to be Him; the Word, Immanuel whose full measure brought life and immortality to light through the gospel.[2]

We don't like or choose garden-experiences for ourselves. We prefer that our religious heroes do the hard part and leave for us a legacy to be admired and a message to be relayed rather than an example to follow. Perhaps we should revise our thinking. If a year's worth of required pandemic distancing does not give us pause and present an opportunity to kneel before the Father in Getheseminian humility we are missing and have missed a tremendous opportunity.

If we were able, despite the violence of interruption and arrest, to debrief Jesus as He completed His garden vigil my guess is that we would be shocked at how sanguine it left Him. Rather than seeing Gethsemane as a wasted chance to give final instructions to His slumbering disciples He saw it as a chance to once again commune with the Father about the mission upon which He was now taking the final steps.

Loneliness is of course a matter of perspective. Loneliness is a matter of focus. Jesus, at the cusp of the cross did not really have time to focus on His loneliness. There in the garden He was not only in intimate conversation with the Father He was also

2. "and which now has been manifested through the appearing of our Savior Christ Jesus, who abolished death and brought life and immortality to light through the gospel," (2 Timothy 1:10 ESV)

surrounded, in a figurative sense, by the fallen masses of forsaken souls whose redemption would be accomplished by His selfless sacrifice. His disciples slept but eternity wept with wonder at the sacrificial humility of the Creator-God who had, in the person of the Son taken on human flesh for the specific purpose of enduring this very night. He became flesh to face down the adversary, suffer the cross, and conquer the grave. Alone? No. We were all there in one way or another filling His thoughts and being whispered in His prayers.

The task for today's Kingdom focused disciples is to enflesh, enlarge, and expand His example in a world which has felt the twin stressors of pandemic disease and political fanaticism. We must be the Church kneeling in the Garden not to abandon the world to Hell, resigned to its fallen, forsaken fate, but praying to act in strength for its redemption when the storm of quarantine breaks and the fractured world is finished with shallow political solutions insufficient to address what is clearly a Spiritual problem. We must emerge stronger. We must come out of our homes prepared. We must face the coming years, uncertain as they may be, with the same focus which allowed the meek Lamb of God to lay low for a time that He might awake in conquest three days. later.

If Jesus could pray through the garden gloom and fulfill His purpose perhaps you and I can go through sequestration, quarantine, and social distancing not only determined to survive, but empowered to thrive. We are nearly on the other side. We do not know what the "new normal" will look like. We have not fully mourned the dead nor have we absorbed the impact of profound social and economic change. Jesus knew what He was facing. He understood it would be painful yet that the afterwards would be worth it for the salvation that it would work and the completeness it would bring. Such confidence should be our goal. Whatever lies before us we, like Jesus, should face it with this purposeful resolve: not my way, not my will, not my wants, not my wishes, not my worries-not me, nor mine-but yours. Your will. Your way. Until we arrive at that place perhaps, we should remain alone in the garden with the whisper of the Spirit in our ear, the words of scripture in our hearts, and the prayer of Jesus on our lips

3

Alone on the Tree

The Psalmist saw but did not understand
What it would mean to be
Broken
Alone
seemingly forsaken
Bloodied
Beaten
Unbowed.

Isaiah too glimpsed the pain so gory
He knew the cost
But not the story.
He envisioned the pain
But not the gain
Which whip
And lance and tree would gain.

In shadows only did they see
That the last time
Jesus would lie
Alone

Would be that moment
Before the angels who came to
Shout the news
Shouldered the stone
As their master
Shoved away death.

A FAMILIAR STORY

ONLY CHRISTMAS HAS A greater hold on Christian imagination than does the passion of Jesus. Doubtless this is because the celebrations surrounding Advent season and Christmas are filled with more immediate "comfort and joy"(to quote the Carol) than we commonly associate with executions.

While the mystery of incarnation is key to the full narrative of the Gospels, it is in at least one sense, the means to an end. The Word stepped into human history so that "God with us" could take His place among us and become in word and deed *the Lamb of God that takes away the sin of the world!*[1] It only seems natural to think of any individual's birth as well as the other highlights of their biography in considering the nature and timing of their death. If this is how we understand history as a tale told regarding the careers of "great men" then this is never more true than it is of Jesus. Some have called the Gospels themselves "passion stories with long introductions" relegating all prior episodes as, in some way, commentary on the cross story. While that maybe a slight exaggeration, it is only slight, inasmuch as each Gospel devotes more space to the passion than any other single episode.

Beyond that, the week-to-week intentional behavior of the Church has always placed the cross and resurrection at the center of its communal life of worship. Even during those seasons of the year where preaching focuses on ethical, eristic, evangelistic, or developmental spirituality, weekly communion reclines us in the upper room with the disciples then flings us to our knees at the

---

1. John 1.29

foot of the cross. Baptizing members into the local and catholic body of the Faithful brings us into an intimate, inclusive participation in the resurrection. Yes, even during Christmas observances themselves there is a clear and well-worn path which leads from the cradle to the cross.

Two of the four Canonical Gospels have nothing to say about Jesus' birth and little information to contribute to understanding His background. In that sense the Gospels are not really biographies in a way that makes sense to our modern sensibilities. We don't know what it was like, though imagination imagines that it does, to grow up in Nazareth, to apprentice as a contractor with Joseph, to worship in Synagogue with the family. We know very little about His childhood, youth, teen-age years. Jesus spiritual formation is largely a mystery to us. Biographical details which the modern mind craves are entirely lacking. We find no juicy tidbits or family drama. We don't know what games Jesus and His brothers played or what role the laborer family may or may not have played in the great architectural and building projects undertaken at Sepphoris, Caesarea, or Tiberias.

In short while we know Jesus, the Jesus we know is the Jesus He Himself chose to reveal and the Jesus who became the foundation character of our mutual faith. Our faith is personal because Jesus did not present Himself as an abstract divine figure. He became as we are. He walked like we walk, communicated in a geographically determined dialect, learned to worship in His localized ancestral fashion, and celebrated the feasts and fasts which defined formative Judaism.

We know Him. We know His story. The Biblical account(s) of what He said and did form not only the doctrinal foundation upon which the Christian Church in all its catholic, distributed tribes is built but also contributed the broader cultural and social context of what, despite the oriental location of His earthly life, became the Western tradition.

So, yes, we know the story. Even those who do not call upon the name of Jesus in faith for salvation have been influenced by the biblical narrative of Passion week. Those for whom Easter is nothing more than a quaint kiddies celebration with colored eggs and chocolate know that at the heart of this Spring celebration is the Christian story of the death, burial, and resurrection of Jesus.

How culture in general, and the Church in particular orients itself to familiar stories frames and empowers those stories. A culture inclined to marginalize everything which cannot be known empirically will look at even its most formative stories with skepticism. The renowned NT Scholar Rudolf Bultman once commented to the effect that "no one who has ever turned on an electric light can reasonably believe in the Biblical world of miracles." Herr Bultman would be shocked at the current crop of metaphysical, supranatural, miraculous, inexplicable, and mysterious phenomena which are currently believed to be true. The Postmodern scientific age may be the most credulous in human history. Our experience during the COVID-19 crisis has provided a stark lesson in how easily Postmodern people can be bamboozled.

- The quasi-religious Qanon cult asserts that there exists a shadow conspiracy of baby-stealing, blood sucking-communist leaning elitists who are trying to secure one-world domination.

- The COVID-19 virus (pick your favorite nonsense theory, is a bio-weapon, can be transmitted by 5G technology, is a hoax.)

- Anti-vax adherents assert that current vaccine efforts are attempts to insert a microchip in the entire world population.

- One of the world's richest men, a great entrepreneur of our time-upon test-launching a space launch vehicle . . . included as payload one of his advanced electric vehicles, carrying a space suit clad mannequin as a passenger.

- Yetis, Sasquatches, aliens, and zombies dominate the airwaves, with little distinction between fiction, documentary, and "reality."

A culture which jettisons faith in the resurrection of Jesus for endless fascination with zombies and vampires has perhaps lost perspective. It is unsettling to think that the time-honored expectation of the coming again of Jesus is thought passe but a heightened expectation for contact with alien intelligences is considered cutting-edge, culturally acceptable science.

Like all familiar stories, including those from the Bible that we have examined so far, familiarity can breed either contempt or contemplation. Contempt for one kind of story often comes at the embrace of another story; even when it is less plausible than the one now abandoned. Story can be myth or mystery. Story can feed faith, or it can be twisted to foment fecklessness and become the butt of some kind of cultural joke in which the naive in society worship and the cultured just take the day off.

One thing which can be hardly denied is the durability of these stories of Christmas and Easter. The Key element is that these stories greatest impact is not cultural but spiritual. Before they changed communities these stories changed lives. Before the Church assumed a leading role in the crumbling of the Roman Empire it first assumed a redemptive role through deeds expressing the loving-kindness of God in Christ Jesus. Before restructuring society there was revival. I do not expect that Discovery Channel specials about Bigfoot or in-depth CNN reports about the intellectual oddities of Qanon will have the same impact on culture. If you do, it might be a good idea to stop reading right now.

Stories have impact. Familiar Scriptures carve their message deeply into our hearts and our minds contributing to the formation of our spiritual character. Yes, we need to carefully and deliberately exegete the stories which have formed us; be they Biblical, cultural, social, historical, or political. There are times when our conclusions about a given story may, perhaps, disappoint us. There are other times when we will find that, despite our best efforts the heart of the story, the very parts which are most transformative elude our capacity to understand. It may be that incarnation, the Godhead, and the operative nature of Jesus' passion fall into that category. It is then that we realize that what we might lack in empirical knowledge comes alive in transformative relationship.

So, how we approach this familiar story both impacts our relationship to Jesus and is impacted *by* our relationship to Jesus.

Faithful Christians began to tell, retell, and preach this story in a hostile environment. In the book of Acts we read how this story defined the message and mission of the early Church. The mission was just beginning, and the story of the cross was front and center. When we broaden our thinking to encompass the Epistles which record the unfolding of Christian doctrine; we find that it all emerges from the nexus of cross and tomb. The unity and clarity of this story told and retold in ever expanding social and cultural contexts and its impact, its tramsforming power continues to stagger the imagination of even the most faithful. Everything we read in those texts occurred in an atmosphere of misunderstanding, repression, opposition, violence, and hostility. Yet, the emerging church, constantly threatened with extermination, defined the faith which even today sustains the worldwide church. The life and ministry of the Church, crystallized in an environment of hate and despite that hate the Church fashioned a message of love.

What explains this durable, determined faith? The story of the cross carried by Jesus informs the story of the cross(es) carried by you and me as we faithfully follow Him. So yes, celebrate Christmas, celebrate the Word becoming incarnate in that mysterious and dark obscurity. But always conduct that reverent celebration in the shadow of the cross. For it is need for the cross which made incarnation necessary.

> "Matthew 27:33 And when they came to a place called Golgotha (which means Place of a Skull), Matthew 27:34 they offered him wine to drink, mixed with gall, but when he tasted it, he would not drink it. Matthew 27:35 And when they had crucified him, they divided his garments among them by casting lots. Matthew 27:36 Then they sat down and kept watch over him there. Matthew 27:37 And over his head they put the charge against him, which read, "This is Jesus, the King of the Jews." Matthew 27:38 Then two robbers were crucified with him, one on the right and one on the left. Matthew 27:39 And those who passed by derided him, wagging their heads Matthew 27:40 and saying, "You who would destroy the temple and rebuild it in three days, save yourself! If you are the Son of God, come

down from the cross." Matthew 27:41 So also the chief priests, with the scribes and elders, mocked him, saying, Matthew 27:42 "He saved others; he cannot save himself. He is the King of Israel; let him come down now from the cross, and we will believe in him. Matthew 27:43 He trusts in God; let God deliver him now, if he desires him. For he said, 'I am the Son of God.'" Matthew 27:44 And the robbers who were crucified with him also reviled him in the same way.Matthew 27:45 Now from the sixth hour there was darkness over all the land until the ninth hour. Matthew 27:46 And about the ninth hour Jesus cried out with a loud voice, saying, "Eli, Eli, lema sabachthani?" that is, "My God, my God, why have you forsaken me?" Matthew 27:47 And some of the bystanders, hearing it, said, "This man is calling Elijah." Matthew 27:48 And one of them at once ran and took a sponge, filled it with sour wine, and put it on a reed and gave it to him to drink. Matthew 27:49 But the others said, "Wait, let us see whether Elijah will come to save him." Matthew 27:50 And Jesus cried out again with a loud voice and yielded up his spirit." (Matthew 27:33–50 ESV)

I know you know this story. If you are a Christian, it is your heritage of faith. If you are an unbeliever, a non-believer, or an agnostic you grew up in a world in which virtually every philosophical, ethical, political, economic, or social theory was reacting in some way against this story. In this story the whole pathology of human sinfulness is on display. Envy. Greed. Anger. Fear. Derision. Contempt. And Jesus is the object. In this story the best representatives of the human community are silent, and the worst hurl verbal abuse at a naked, bleeding, dying, man.

The story of the cross compounds the thousand papercuts of sin into one final sadistic catastrophe. The entire created order joins in the mourning of heaven as Jesus dies. It is a story, if true which both exalts and diminishes humanity. It elevates us by holding out the prospect that our sinful, destructive tendencies can somehow be brought to heel, if the best among us sacrifices self to accomplish that needed atonement. That is, of course what the NT teaches. We are utterly unable to deal satisfactorily with our own sin, our own alienation from God. The Biblical story beginning in the OT and continuing through the earthly ministry of Jesus is the tale of God's incessant quest to do for us finally and fully what we cannot do for ourselves. This, the passion story, is final-or more accurately-the opening of the final phase of this still-ongoing and unfolding plan.

This story diminishes humanity by reminding us of the lows to which we can continually fall. Jesus did nothing but good and the result was the worst treatment imaginable. No wonder the prophets only knew part of the story. Had they known beforehand the depth of human depravity and the treachery of human rebellion, had they any hint at what God's plan fully entailed, surely they would have in some way objected. Both Psalmist and Isaiah knew, but only in part. They did not, they could not have envisioned that God Himself would suffer so terribly in the tangible form of incarnate Word. They could only see in symbols how the Son would bear the guilt of all our sin. How could they fully understand the beatings? How could they comprehend the torture? How could they imagine the Son of God being tortured, as His saving sacrifice became in actuality what their poetry portrayed; a Lamb eternally marked by the stripes by which we are healed?

Beyond the familiarity we have from reading and enjoying this story as text; this story is symbolically retold every time any Christian of any tribal (denominational) affiliation gathers to consume bread and wine to commemorate it. It is the story that birthed the Church-and at the very center is a naked man being tortured to death to satisfy the ambition of men who could not countenance competition.

Caesar does not share his imperial authority. The priests mistook their ministry as a license to steal. They thought that the temple treasury belonged to those who collected it. Formerly these business-focused High-priests were anointed by God to intercede on behalf of His people with prayer and sacrifice and devotion. Now? Now they were appointed by the Emperor not to balance the account of the people's sins but to balance the accounts of the people's tithes. Tithes to God. Taxes to Caesar. It's all the same when your wealth and privilege are built upon taking a cut. The Pharisees had been relegated to winning hearts and minds- which is generally a euphemism for "we don't have any power." So, they became the most overtly liberal (overbearing, meddling, know-it-alls, and do-gooders) of their co-religionists. Of course, the Temple bankers and the Herodian collaborators were ultra-conservative-the status quo was making them rich! The Pharisees became the party of religious pride. Pride gave way to passion. Passion led them to positions of respect. Which passion also left them vulnerable to paranoia. So, after initial sparring and then teasingly testing Jesus, they quickly realized that they could not win a competition with Jesus. They could not contend with His voice. They could not match His authoritative demeanor. They could not equal His alignment of doctrine and deeds. Like most of us the Pharisees feared most that which was most admirable.

The story of the cross reminds us that every political, social, ethnic, religious, economic, and political interest aligned against Jesus. This is a revealing lesson about formal social and cultural systems as well as ad-hoc grouping of human beings. What is really treasured is what primarily motivates. You will remember that Jesus Himself said basically the same thing. (Where your treasure is . . .) What we can so clearly see in the story is, to use the tried and true (if a bit old-fashioned) biblical phrase; Ox goring is fine—except mine. Go after enough oxen, question the values and virtues of too many of the powerful elites and you will find (to change the metaphor) your goose cooked.

So these disparate groups put aside their own, very real differences, and worked together on the common cause of crucifying the man with whom they could not compete. No man can box with God and win. And, despite His best efforts, they never got the message that in seeing Jesus, they were seeing God. In confronting Jesus, they were confronting God. In dismissing Jesus, they were dismissing God. Jesus did not die despite His goodness (which is the common, all too human assumption). Jesus died because of His goodness. It was because the expanding, collusive, corrupting power of Empire was most threatened not by the rabble (which

Rome fed and entertained) but by the righteous one. The rabble, the mob, the crowd—they can be easily bought off, as can narcissistic disciples. The righteous Son of God, the exemplary Son of Man could not be bought off or shut out. The only way to silence Him, so they thought, was to do so permanently. The rest of the story, reminds us exactly how wrong they proved to be.

One of the central contributions of the 21c is ubiquitous connectivity. Even when we remained all alone in our socially-distanced bubbles, while the plague ravaged our world and we feared for life and livelihood, even then we were able to call, chat, video, zoom, and share. Clearly the "alone" we were experiencing during the pandemic was different, not only in degree, but in kind from the alienation experienced by Jesus on that long ago day on that far away hill.

On that stage not only was His physical body naked, His heart and His mind and His spirit were exposed to heaven and earth. He was exposed for heaven to mourn and for earth to scorn. He was displayed before friend and foe; seemingly powerless evidently despondent. Alone but watched. For there were eyes upon Him. He was silent while angry voices shouted around Him. Calloused hands mishandled Him and secured Him. Gloating grins gazed upon the Galilean finally certain that in this moment, amongst this mob they had triumphed. Yet, in the midst of that crowd of tormenters, torturers and toadies, on that very stage to which He had aimed His whole life, in that place, before all creation. He. Was. Alone.

A DISTURBING DEVELOPMENT

With the mocking of the thieves in His ears-He died. Without addressing the charges of the Temple authorities or the scribes, theologians, and popular teachers-He died. Without replying to the insinuations of treason by the emperor's proxy-He died. The first time we hear the outcome of the Cross-story, most of us are shocked. We are raised on stories in which the resolution of the plot, the elimination of the tension is brought full circle by the epitomeatic phrase "they lived happily ever after." The tale of the tree is, neither fairy tale nor nightmare. Like virtually every real human story, and like basically the entire Old Testament, the story of the cross is a realistic tragedy. In the real world the high-priest and his cronies leave the trial and go off to a late brunch, while the Lamb of God whose death was symbolized by every sacrifice offered under the priestly vocation, was led off to a hungry and hopeless death.

At the very heart of the central story of human history is the inescapable fact that the Creator, sustainer of the universe died alone. He who chose to gather a motley group of disciples around His fledgling ministry died without those chosen students present. He who gathered crowds who hung on His every word and cheered for every deed, died alone in the middle of a mob crying out for a vengeance they did not need, against an individual who did not deserve it, for a cause they could not yet understand. That is the heart of the story of the Cross.

Alone again. He had scripture. As He had in the desert He was prepared with the words of Law and Psalm to give Him strength and insight during this darkest moment. Unlike that encounter years before the Adversary was clever enough to keep his mouth shut. Enough had already been said! The charges brought, the accusations made. Now, the liar, having lied it was time to lay low and watch the death of God unfold!

Instead of speaking himself, unable to restrain himself entirely, Satan spoke through proxies that day around the cross. Over and over again the words spoken through others were replete with his favorite themes of excess, ambition, and destruction. He spoke through the voice of Judas' greed and ambition. The clumsy protestation of how he, an innocent man was taken advantage of, thus condemning another innocent man to die alone. The snake surely snickered at that, then whispered the desperate words of self-loathing, torment, and condemnation which led Judas—in his own time and to a far different purpose to also die-ironically and truly-alone.

In much the same way the deceiver spoke through the Sanhedrin, and libeling witnesses, and all those who thought that screaming in a mob would silence the rumbling of their consciences. It is so easy to manipulate the malleable when there is much at stake. Some in the crowd murmured. "Who knows? Perhaps the leaders know something we do not." That is the mystique of elite power in a highly structured society. "Surely they know best. Surely, we can trust them. Of course, they understand the stakes. They must have considered the cost."

A crowded courtroom, a docket filled with fools, liars, hypocrites, hucksters, and hooligans. And they were the judges! And Jesus stood alone! Any who had sought to live according to the standard of the Law the Sanhedrin thought they were applying, though they were in fact denying—those people wanted no part of the proceedings. Excluded from considering the curious case of the one called Christ, Nicodemus and Joseph would emerge later to care for the temporarily lifeless form of the beloved whom they were unable serve in life.

The devil had long prepared for this day. The day he saw as the ultimate opportunity to wreck God's plans and destroy creation. And at the center of it all this day, the one who had come defiantly proclaiming in His own name and on His own terms a peace that Caesar ever promised and never delivered. He promised healing from the ravages of a disease Empire could not even comprehend. Now, on this day and in this place the evil one seemed to have brought the entire machine of redemption to a screeching halt. On this day the Devil duped Empire itself into driving the nails, supplying the soldiers, and wielding the whip. The Father of Lies deluded Pilate himself into writing the sarcastic epitaph over what seemed to be becoming the sorriest of all attempts at salvation. *King of the Jews.* KING OF THE JEWS? King of the Jews hanging on a tree? King of the Jews treated like a criminal? King of the Jews nakedly exposed to the world as a fraud!? King of the Jews? Surrounded not by adoring crowds, not thronged by devoted worshippers. Instead, the King of the Jews surrounded by someone else's soldiers, hearing someone else's curses. Bleeding His own blood.

Holding back His own screams. Choking on the stench of His own bodily filth being released in the throes of torturous death. Not since that sunny day in Eden had the dragon beheld a man more alone, more battered, more forlorn. Not since that day when Lady Eve first felt the deadening knowledge of sin had the Serpent seen someone looking so longingly for the face of God.

He may not have known that anything was amiss but perhaps felt a slight twinge of doubt when Jesus singingly, haltingly, whisperingly spoke. Those around the cross must have thought Jesus was becoming delirious, thirsty, weakened, and raving. As they ran to get the condemned a drink, Satan shivered. He had heard Jesus quote scripture before, on another day when he thought that he had successfully alienated Jesus. On that day the Scriptures rolled from Jesus lips with a power to make the desert spring to life. And now, again, in the throes of death He, sings a Psalm. Satan did not yet know what it meant this day, but He knew that even in death this God-in-Flesh was dangerous enough to destroy all his designs of darkness.

So, Satan had his day and the sun darkened and gloom consumed the land. Jesus alone with God, bowed His head, prayed out His last breath and prepared to have the last laugh.

RESPONSIBLE RESOLUTION

What is the right resolution to what seems to be the central human problem; dying alone? Despite years of selfless ministry by which He endeared Himself to others Jesus hung alone on that final, critical day of His life and ministry. He experienced at that final moment of dreadful despair the same solitary reality of all humans, all life, all creatures. Death eventually stares us all in the face and there is no one there to confront it with us.

Jesus, despite all appearances did not, necessarily see it that way. He understood not only the first line of Psalm 22, which he quoted from the cross, he also understood the rest of the Psalm with its promise of the Father's deliverance, salvation and yes, presence at that moment when breath flees the body.

"For he has not despised or abhorred the affliction of the afflicted, and he has not hidden his face from him, but has heard, when he cried to him. I will tell of your name to my brothers; in the midst of the congregation I will praise you: You who fear the LORD, praise him! All you offspring of Jacob, glorify him, and stand in awe of him, all you offspring of Israel For he has not despised or abhorred the affliction of the afflicted, and he has not hidden his face from him, but has heard, when he cried to him." (Psalm 22:22–24 *ESV*)

The perception of the spectators[2] was that Jesus had been abandoned by the God who He had faithfully served. His disciples, who He had faithfully taught and led were nowhere to be seen. They hid in the margins or stood in solidarity with a few weeping women. Some who were related to Him, and others whose connection to Him was of course, suspect. Otherwise, Jesus went to His cross with few friends. Instead, there were enemies and observers. The mocking and the malevolent. A few broken souls shattered by the experience of seeing their teacher tortured and executed. Jesus expiring in their midst. To a disinterested observer it certainly looked like He was alone in any meaningful or helpful sense of the term. It appears that he has been forsaken by all those whom he loved and who claimed to love him.

However, Jesus knows scripture. His life and ministry were intentional from the pre-incarnational councils of God to the central tenets of his life and teaching. If prior to the cross nothing had happened by accident, then from Jesus' perspective, His resolve at least, had not changed. Even now, as His blood flowed, His life ebbed, and His heart broke the Father was in charge, heaven was in attendance, the divine purposes were being realized.

We who are bounded by mortality and constrained by the fall look at the Cross and see despair. Indeed, there was pain and suffering, brokenness and blood, the reflexive fear of those who courageously face pain and persecution. Yet, there is also victory. John

2. Audience, crowd, gallery, mob? One is at some pains to describe the attitude of the onlookers. Perhaps the crowd crowded around the cross did so with mixed motives. Some hostile, some sympathetic, some in shock.

tells us that his final words were not words of despair, defeat, or dereliction-but words of victory. *When Jesus had received the sour wine, he said, "It is finished," and he bowed his head and gave up his spirit.*[3] How could Jesus, even Jesus be so confident in the hour of deepest darkness? He knew the promise of the third day, He knew that the promise of restoration, the promise of resurrection was no empty boasting. It was the plan all along. It was God's purpose the whole time. The only responsible resolution to the shameful shattering of His life, the only faithful action was to submit and await the Father's promise.

Surely Satan was amused at the spectacle. Generations had lived and died; millennia had passed. Every nuance of his adversarial skill had been used to deflect and distract the few fumbling faithful feckless sons and daughters of Adam who had tried to keep faith with their creator. Did he do it from spite, anger, malice, or amusement? Likely each attitude motivated him then, and continue to motivate him now. Even in the biblical story the pathetic attempts of faithful people to avoid sin and to keep from breaking faith are multiplied. And here, at the last, with God incarnate walking among His "own" He was able to turn one of the intimates of the Son, to compromise him to entice him, ultimately manipulate him into aiding and abetting the destruction he had intended for this moment when God himself came to rescue the race.

So, Satan had the last laugh. The snake snickered. The accuser guffawed. The irresponsible, weakened, incarnate Son-had failed! Then the lingering laughter of Lucifer turns to dust in his mouth at the awakening of God's Son and the echoing shout of resurrection heard throughout the kingdoms, empires, and principalities of the fallen world.

As Satan's laughter turned to despair: Angels giggled.

We have suffered plague, pandemic, political panic, and very real pain. The question we must ask in our time and at our place is quite simple. Whose laughter do you hear when you lay your head down at night? Is it the sarcastic sneer of Satan who looks upon pain and suffering as his tools of torment to distract God's

---

3. John 19.30

creation from the opportunity for salvation and wholeness? Or do you close your eyes and hear the Angels? Do you hear them sing and shout? Do you hear them giggle and weep? Do you hear the cry of the rising Son of God-

> *"Fear not, I am the first and the last, and the living one. I died, and behold I am alive forevermore, and I have the keys of Death and Hades."* (Revelation 1:17–18 ESV)

He reacted in the only responsible way that our incarnate creator-God could possibly respond. He rose from the dead by the power of the Father to bring life and immortality to light. How should we react considering the dignity and responsibility expected of us by the Son our Savior who suffered so much in passing through the grave to redeem us?

> *"Therefore, as you received Christ Jesus the Lord, so walk in him, rooted and built up in him and established in the faith, just as you were taught, abounding in thanksgiving." (Colossians 2:6–7 ESV)*

We are tempted to whine, equivocate, wander, and wish that things were different, that we were not called to discipline and cross-carrying. That is not the gospel for which Jesus suffered and died. That is not the gospel which the Apostles and their companions in the embryonic church proclaimed. That is not the word preached in Jerusalem, Rome, or Antioch and that is not the Gospel I will preach in Grayville.

> *"Consider him who endured from sinners such hostility against himself, so that you may not grow weary or faint-hearted." (Hebrews 12:3 ESV)*

Jesus went to the cross. His conquest of death has provided to you not only an example of how to encounter and overcome the silent oppression of loneliness but how to conquer your questioning fear, teaching you to serve him with gladness.

The times always seem more desperate than they are. We sometimes feel more alone than we should. This is not just pious speculation speaking to itself in reassuring tones, oblivious to the actual circumstances in our world. It is not wishful whistling in the dark. No, faith carries us out of lonliness and isolation to that special place where we can see the face and hear the voice of God. Jesus on the cross did not let circumstances dictate His response or diminish His determined faith.

Every human individual, every person made in the image of God was made for eternal fellowship with the Father. This fellowship sometimes only emerges after purging solitude. Often, it is in that very solitude, that we are best situated to appreciate His presence. When we resent the isolation which drives us into the presence of God, we forsake one of the foundations which forms faithful character.

I have not spent time in these meditations considering saints from the Old Testament who walked the path of solitude but there are many. Abraham's path from Ur through Haran to the promised land is an example. He was accompanied by many—yet it was in solitude that he chose to listen and respond to the I AM. Isaac mourned his mother alone in his tent. Rich as he was it was not until he saw his bride and beheld his future that he began to emerge into his patriarchal duty. Jacob? Alone with God on the bank of a creek contemplating his own continual history of chicanery, bamboozlement, and graft he finally realized that God could not be fooled and that sometimes faith is the only way out and the only way up.

We will spend many months perhaps even years reflecting upon social-distancing, quarantine, and isolation. Some will try and hide in impermeable tents seeking to exclude eternal questions. Others will see this year as nothing but a huge social experiment of governmental overreach and over reaction. Still others will confront God and hold Him accountable for the havoc wrought whilst withholding from Him any devotion. Though seemingly alone with your thoughts, your prayers, your reflections, your insights, your fears, and your resentments—you are joined by everyone else sharing the same circumstances. Some will come to the cross only to shake their fist and to blame the Christ they otherwise ignore. Others will come to the cross for answers to gnawing questions.

Some of us, hopefully all who wear the name of Jesus, will come to the cross because we know that the solitary, naked, bleeding, dying figure there, won the ultimate battle over all forms of our fallen isolation. What questions will you bring, what doubt will you abandon, when you contemplate His lonely, dying, figure at the foot of the Cross?

Let us close our solemn time around the cross with this observation. Some have been taken by this awful disease. While we were fighting a new and unforeseen plague others fell to the common afflictions, old age, diabetes, heart disease, hatred, happenstance, and cancer. If you are reading these words that is not your fate. If you are still with me on this journey of reflection it is because you have survived (at least the first phase) of this journey. If you are reading these words and wear the name of Christ you are called to embrace the responsible service first demonstrated by the all-conquering Son. He rose that you might live. He conquered that you, like Him, might live a life poured out for many. It is shocking how many Christians assert their rights and decry "mistreatment" who then bow their knees to Jesus—the crucified—expecting affirmation for the very selfish frame of mind which made the cross necessary in the first place. The only responsible reaction? Die to self so that we might rise in loving service to others through the empowering Spirit of the one who now holds the keys to death and the grave.

4

Singing Alone in the City Jail

The walls of my house
Are not a jail.
We don't social distance
Cause we can't make bail.

Some cry for freedom
When they already are
But they don't think it counts
If they can't drink in a bar.

And they'd never submit
To objectionable rules
Of tyrants and rogues
Laws are just tools.

Yet faithful believers
The freest of free
Still must submit
Though we may not agree.

So, Silas and Paul
Were thrown in a cell
They took their licks
Did not bicker or yell.

For doing their duty
Not any wrong
They responded with joy
Filled the jail with their song.

A FAMILIAR STORY

THERE IS NO LONELINESS quite like the loneliness which is entirely avoidable. Even then, Paul was not entirely alone. One of the members of his team, Silas, was with him in the jail where he was securely fixed in stocks. They did not have to be there. It certainly impacted Paul's state of mind to know that they were there in that cell due to the pursuit of mission. In a sense, Silas' presence was collateral damage. Since this episode is taken from one of the "We" sections of Acts clearly Paul's entire evangelistic team was participating in the worship gatherings and ministry in Philippi though only Paul and Silas were taken into custody. Presumably they were more active or perceived to be a greater threat than Luke and any others who may have been present.

During the current pandemic some have raised the specter of governmental meddling and various species of persecution or at least, harassment. One of the ironies of Twenty-Twenty is the sense, that despite the governments of the world being ill prepared for what happened, their responses should be evaluated as if they had long-standing plans which should have accounted for every eventuality and considered the feelings of every sub-constituency they served.

Athletic stadiums were closed, and it was an economic disaster. Restaurants were closed and livelihoods thereby lost. Hospitals could not perform elective surgeries and they too felt the sting of economic hardship. The social and fraternal clubs were closed, and members spoke out about violations of rights. And churches could not gather for public worship. To which the response was anger, disillusionment and claims of persecution. Earliest Christianity produced courageous martyrs. Twenty-First century Christianity produced entitled whiners. Interestingly, those who encounter real, bona-fide, malicious, destructive, persecution tend to be more sanguine about the circumstances they experience and focused on the outcome of their testimony to faith. Which discussion brings us back to Paul.

Paul's life seems to have come, in a sense, full circle. After all, he had first encountered Christians from the other side of law and order. Before the Damascus Road experience, prior to his conversion, before his Apostolic mission, before the foundation of churches and the writing of letters, before all that—Paul was in the business of doing to others what had now been done to him. Maybe, despite the discomfort, he chuckled at the irony.

He came to the colonial city of Philippi to begin Christ's conquest of Europe. For those of us of European descent it seems odd to consider that up until this time the Gentiles in the Church were most likely of Asian ancestry and that they were still a minority. The center of gravity for Paul's ministry at this point was still Asia Minor. Certainly, by this time, the churches he had founded were already beginning the penetration of the regions of which they were typically the chief cities. This process would take time and eventually the Church would flourish. That was in the future.

As his foundation churches began the organic expansion which led to world-wide dominance Paul transitioned to opening the next broad field. His plan, in retrospect, seems to have been a basic movement west accompanied with return visits to Antioch, where it all began. Now this mission brought him to Philippi where he found a small Jewish prayer group; as he always did He engages that group in conversation, lecturing, Biblical study and eventually evangelistic preaching.

Lydia and her household became the first truly European outpost of the Church founded by Jesus and extended by the efforts of first century missionaries like Paul. However, (you surely knew the other shoe would drop) Philippi was unlike the other cities where Paul had founded congregations faithful to Jesus. Philippi was a Roman *Colonia*. The first citizens had been Roman soldiers paroled from Civil War who had been granted property and status in this new outpost of Empire. Given their background the inhabitants of Philippi were rather strict in their enforcement of imperial-style law and order. Additionally, they were embedded in the Empire's sprawling Pagan-Economic nexus. The Roman empire used conquest to further its economic ends. Its economic ends were furthered by social stability. Social stability was insured by a combination of top-down Imperial enforcement and local cooperative government. That fragile, coalition approach to Empire required religion-paganism-in all its silly, superstitious, strangeness to be the glue that held the various constituents together.

Jews like Lydia[1] were welcomed in pagan society so long as they did not disturb the peace and played their role in expanding and extending the economic system. Paul was himself a craftsman, so he understood the combination of factors which made the empire function. As a Jew he was a benefactor of the many privileges which had been granted to both the Jewish Nation and the Synagogue both in Judea and the dispersion.

He was also a central actor in the way that the fragile balance was being upset. His targeted travels and long-term purpose of preaching the Gospel of Jesus Christ throughout the empire had first brought him into direct conflict with various configurations of Jewish authority figures who disagreed with his interpretation both of the Old Testament in general, and his particular application of the Old Testament to the life, ministry, and passion of Jesus. It goes without saying that his Jewish disputants disagreed with his conclusions about Jesus' divine origins, the scandal of the cross and his insistence that his very Apostleship was contingent on his meeting with the resurrected Christ.

---

1. Presumably unmarried, but also possibly in a mixed marriage either of which explains why no husband is mentioned and the way she made her livelihood is emphasized.

It is easy to cast the disagreements in which Paul and other early Christians found themselves entangled as nothing more than theological disagreements which simply got out of hand. While this is satisfying to a world conditioned by twenty centuries of Christian preaching and which prides itself on tolerant attitudes toward religious difference it does not really do justice to the composition of the ancient world nor to the confluence of all the aforementioned factors which contributed to the totalizing social experiment which was the Roman empire.

For example, paganism was not really, to our way of understanding, theological at all. In fact, most of us would not recognize paganism as particularly religious. A pagan could make his or her sacrifices and direct his or her life according to the tenets of Stoicism, Epicureanism, or the emerging demi-philosophy of Neo-Platonism. It did not really make any difference. Pagan religion was almost entirely about performance.

Of course, by this time formative, Judaism was making the transformation from a sacrifice driven cult to a theologically driven outgrowth of the Synagogue. This transformation was occurring at the very moment when Paul was traversing the Empire proclaiming the universal Lordship of the risen Christ. And now the conflict between Church and Synagogue was accelerating, largely due to Paul's intentional, focused efforts at global expansion.

After the conference recorded in Acts 15 it was becoming apparent that Gentiles would be admitted to the Church without first becoming Jews. This did not sit well with certain elements in the Church and fared even worse with those who did not agree that Jesus was the Christ and that the Gospel of the resurrection best explained the Hebrew Scriptures.

Consequently, Paul in Philippi was a man who was marshalling his efforts for battle on two fronts. Theologically and socially, he would be in contention with formative Judaism. Religiously, politically, and economically his foe would be Imperial Paganism. After all the intervening centuries it sometimes escapes contemporary Christians just how difficult this balancing act was for Paul.

Formative Judaism and Earliest Christianity we must re-member, were sibling religious outlooks each of which sprang out of the foment of 2nd Temple Judaism. Each saw itself as the true heir of the faith traditions of Abraham, as further refined by the Sinai-revelation of Moses, extended by the prophets, and the other worship or wisdom focused traditions found in the Hebrew Bible. Even in the lifetime of Jesus there were differences of opinion which moved beyond the scope of mere differences in theologi-cal opinion or practice. And as the empire had its confluence of economic, political, cultural, and practical concerns so did the two competitors for interpretive preeminence regarding the Hebrew scriptures and traditions.

Formative Judaism consisted of multiple exegetical outlooks which were really refinements of prior competing traditions which, having emerged in the Hasmonean and Hellenistic periods of Ju-dean history, ossified in opposition to one another under Roman rule. On a continuum some were more violent (the "zealots") oth-ers less (the Essenes.) Some of the groups in and around Jerusalem chose to work hand-in-glove with the governing authorities be they Romans specifically or their collaborative toadies. Formative Judaism, specifically the Pharisaic branch which would further evolve into Rabbinic Judaism, and finally into the Judaism(s) we know today was the branch from which Paul was descended spiri-tually and the version in which he learned to read and interpret scripture. Like any closely related yet estranged groups "Jews" and "Christians" were antagonistic-more because of what they shared theologically than what they rejected. They agreed on the extent of the Hebrew Scriptures but not exegesis. They accepted the in-spiration of scripture but not its interpretation. They agreed on resurrection as an abstract principle but not as specifically demon-strated by Jesus. Their prime disagreement, both while Jesus was present, and later with the emerging Church, was on the nature and authority of tradition.

Jesus was the crux because many of the Jews which Paul and other missionaries addressed were "vulnerable" to the Churches reading of the scripture. They agreed on so much that really it came down to deciding for or against Jesus. Once Jesus was understood to be resurrected Lord that entailed a hermeneutical shift which essentially answered questions about Canon and Tradition. Ultimately (at least from the perspective of those of us who wear the name of Christ) the reason the Church triumphed, the reason the Synagogue was so jealous was Jesus Himself, whose claims to Lordship on the one hand and resurrection on the other, made His gospel appealing in contexts both Jewish and Pagan. It is difficult to argue the intricacies and minutia of theology with the followers of someone who is persistently and stubbornly no longer dead.

So, as Paul and his team of collaborators, scribes, secretaries, trainees, and hangers-on made their way throughout the Empire they were constantly shadowed by contentious groups whose strategy was to demean the message by besmirching the messenger. Some of these figures shared allegiance to Jesus but rejected the compromise arrived at in Acts 15 whereby Gentiles were accepted into the Church as Gentiles. Others did not share any faith in Jesus and attacked the hermeneutic process as well as the missionary procedure of Paul.

Everywhere Team Paul went they were required to debate and defend their faith in Jesus, their interpretation of the Hebrew Scriptures, (often relying upon the Septuagint, the common Greek version as their primary witness thereof) their methodology, and goals. While this was likely an exhausting way to do business it had the long-term unintended consequence (through their interlocutors at least) of helping the earliest Church clarify its essential questions, refine its methods, delineate its aims in interpreting scripture and, systematize the rapidly evolving teaching of the Church. It also required Paul and those around him to think quickly, accurately, courageously, and creatively on their feet.

Religiously[2], economically and socially Paul and his contingent would also be in contention with Empire. As with the

2. Again, Paganism was Religious . . . but not Theological. Everything about Paganism from the names shared among the Gods and Goddesses, the games and festivals, the shrines and temples-it was all always in flux. So long as Rome's genius was honored, and the treasure flowed ever upward to Rome.

prevalent understanding of Judaism, our perspective on Rome, its empire, political system, social theory, and religious history is far too dependent on projecting our own world and worldviews into the ancient world.

Contemporary conceptions of politics are typified by clear, often polarized distinctions. Modern political and economic theories are based on an Enlightenment understanding of the relationships between autonomous human beings and macro-autonomous governing structures. Popularly elected representative governments, to our way of thinking, express the epitome of political organization. These forms of government are most often found embodied in constitutions which call for separation or concentration of powers.[3] These are constitutional systems in which individualistic concerns are adjudicated by autonomous individuals who, because of wealth, standing, popularity, or ability are selected to represent other autonomous individuals in what is in essence, a process of negotiation with respect to distributing rights, property, opportunity, and sovereignty. Whew. That is a long, complex definition, the purpose of which was to clarify that our world and the Roman world are entirely different.

Even in discussing Enlightenment and Post-Enlightenment examples of Empire it is abundantly clear that our politics is different, our economics has different goals, our conception of the place of the individual in society has a different focus, and the structures created to sustain our order have different orienting values.

Rome had been a Republic. Real Romans were always nostalgic for the old days. For some the Empire would always be a historical anomaly which spoiled the fortune spilled upon the glory of Italy. The distinction on the impoverished lower classes was lost. Starvation is starvation and exploitation painful regardless of the structures in place. The difference between Imperial and Republican Rome was essentially the same as that between Soviet Russia and Post-Soviet Russa—none. Thieves are thieves and nostalgia

---

3. In the systems of representative governance found in the American and British systems respectively.

never seems to be powerful enough to lure those who escape totalitarian clutches to longingly return.

Our understanding of Imperial Rome is often too simplistic and too complex, all at the same time. Rome was a complicated society before they seized the mantle of Empire[4] from the descendants and inheritors of Alexander. Rome absorbed the governing institutions, structures, alliances, and understandings which had gone before, infusing them with the practical sense of Roman law while continuing the noble and ancient practices of graft and corruption. In the first century Rome was still evolving. It had been an empire for less than a century. Some citizens longed for republican days of old. Still others understood that the hunger for imperial preeminence required and drove an ever-expanding empire. So, Rome grew. Conquering territory whilst being conquered by foreign culture. Achieving political preeminence at the expense of religious syncretism. Rome found very early in its imperial history that most pagans were easily placated by promises of continued "religious freedom." So long as the local Pantheon gave preeminence to the gods of Rome and the genius of the Roman state. Paganism itself was a logical outgrowth of human hubris and the lust for conquest and cultural imperialism. If the God's are many, if plural worship is admirable—even advisable, the more Gods the better!

And though we in contemporary society have arrived at an uneasy truce with the notion that Religion should accrue wealth to itself there was no such scruple in the ancient world. Temples were the banks of the day! It was in the giving of gifts, offering of sacrifices, the selling of idols and trinkets and souvenirs and monuments that wealth accrued to temples and thereby to the

---

4. I understand Empire to be that Trans-national constellation of the Nations in opposition to Kingdom. The Babylonians, Persians, Greeks came before Rome. Traditionally we would say they "had Empire" or controlled Empire. To my way of thinking they were themselves had by Empire . . . controlled by the broader satanic impulse to oppose God's rule. This impulse, which was first sighted in the Bible in Genesis 3, becomes a totalizing oppositional force in Genesis 11, where on the plains of Shinar the notion of fully ascendant human culture and society first flourished and then foundered.

cities wherein they were located and thereby to the Empire which taxed the entire structure of what we naively call worship and piously describe as "religious."

Politics. Economics. Religion. For Rome these were simply different descriptions of the same thing. This can be said of most ancient or at least pre-modern societies yet those of us raised in the Enlightenment or Post-enlightenment traditions need to constantly remind ourselves that it is entirely possible that our culture of neat division between religion, ethics, philosophy, science, economics, politics, race, sex/gender-is perhaps the historic outlier. In fact there are many commonalities between the Roman world and our current postmodern culture.

So, this familiar Bible story recounts historical developments that could have been foreseen but which are often overlooked in our sanctimonious rush to find the "spiritual" or devotional angle of the text. Yet this story will erupt in a spiritual dislocation unlike anything the world had ever seen before. Paul and those with him will begin a revolution against two of the central defining features of the ancient world. Judaism will be dismissed as the revelatory force of the Creator God because of its rejection of Jesus. Judaism's approach to the Hebrew Bible will be superseded by the hermeneutic of Emerging Christianity. Paul and his successors, will view the entire world as their mission field, will fearlessly proclaim faith in Jesus. At the very same time Paul will open a second front calling into question the entire intellectual, spiritual, and social focus of Empire exposing its pretense of peace, unity, and plenty as an empty promise. Every ox gored. Every pretense exposed. Every untruth unveiled. Every idol destroyed. That is what motivated Paul. That is context for the conflict we read about. A conflict which began in the marketplace, of a city set along a river.

A DISTURBING DEVELOPMENT

Now that we have properly reviewed the ideology of Empire and have a better understanding of how we should contrast it with formative Judaism we can arrive at a better picture of what happened in Philippi and why it was so significant.

On the one hand we can surmise that the Jewish community in Philippi was small. There was no hall in which the Synagogue met. In fact, with Lydia being mentioned as the chief person in the small worshiping community it appears likely that there was not the required number of 10 Jewish men available to conduct Synagogue worship. Still, they met and they prayed. Because formative Judaism had been evolving in diaspora communities since the Assyrian conquest of the Northern Kingdom (Israel) in the 8th century BC, Jewish communities were durable and adaptive when it came to time, place, and organization for worship. Paul found them, joined them, preached to them, persuaded them, and ultimately baptized them into Christ. This was his habit. This was his method. He was clearly good at this process of meeting and teaching and the Lord blessed him with the same sort of success which he had in Asia Minor.

To our mind what happened to Paul next, the event which resulted in his involuntary social distancing was unconscionable. He did a good deed. As a spiritual man he exercised as much restraint as he could before taking matters into his own hands and solving a problem that was becoming a very public spectacle.

> 16 *As we were going to the place of prayer, we were met by a slave girl who had a spirit of divination and brought her owners much gain by fortune-telling. 17 She followed Paul and us, crying out, "These men are servants of the Most High God, who proclaim to you the way of salvation." 18 And this she kept doing for many days. Paul, having become greatly annoyed, turned and said to the spirit, "I command you in the name of Jesus Christ to come out of her." And it came out that very hour. Acts 16:16–18 (ESV)*

Here is where those cultural differences between Imperial Rome and contemporary Western society function as essential lenses through which to view the events. Nothing was "just" religious. Nothing was "just" politics. Nothing was "just" economics. If we were to view the modern world as a Venn graph the three circles— politics, economics and religion would intersect. For some specific nations or regions one or the other would predominate and the extent of overlap would similarly fluctuate. In the ancient world the three circles would be directly on top of each other. Everything was wholly involved with everything else. What seems outrageous to us was perfectly normal to them.

We need to constantly ask ourselves "how normative is *our* experience?" When we judge "primitive" cultures either anthropologically or biblically how can we be sure that we are being as objective as we can possibly be? What if we are the outliers? The fact of the matter is that the Enlightenment understanding of man and his place in the world was innovative and experimental. The jury is still out on whether it is a success or failure.

So it is as a Jew, a Christian convert, an educated Hellenist, a Pharisee, and a Roman citizen that Paul finds himself locked up for a crime which culturally, has almost always been thought of as a commercial or economic crime in which Paul interfered with the "property" of someone else. Our modern sensibilities are shocked by what we understand to be an invasion of Paul's personal religious privacy rights. Which religion? Which privacy? What of the others involved in the affair?

> "And when they had brought them to the magistrates, they said, "These men are Jews, and they are disturbing our city. They advocate customs that are not lawful for us as Romans to accept or practice." The crowd joined in attacking them, and the magistrates tore the garments off them and gave orders to beat them with rods. And when they had inflicted many blows upon them, they threw them into prison, ordering the jailer to keep them safely. Having received this order, he put them into the inner prison and fastened their feet in the stocks. (Acts 16:20–24ESV)

In the contextual matrix of a racially mixed, culturally diverse, religiously plural imperial community the response of the authorities would seem entirely appropriate. One individual has had their property rights permanently injured. His property rights in an enslaved, (probably) sexually exploited minor-offensive as they are to us-were perfectly normal in that context. The religious dimension should not be ignored either. The specific economic gain this particular slave girl brought to her masters was only possible because she was spirit possessed, that is endowed with what they understood to be pagan and cultic sensitivity to the spirit world. To her owner this spiritual sensitivity enabled his profit motive. Paul healed him right out of a gift that kept on giving. And in true imperial style it was a gift that was his to exploit in the person of another individual weaker than himself.

Of course he reacted as the offended party! He was likely a Roman citizen and as such would understand his rights before the bar and expect them to be upheld. He likely looked down on individuals like Paul who were making their way from the eastern parts of the empire polluting the Roman world with new ideas, new gods, new religions, new cultural expectations. Did he think in terms of renewed Roman greatness? Did he express his anger at what the empire had become through the continual extension of the Roman peace? Perhaps he was fed up with continual immigration. Maybe he was a Roman patriot, a seasoned culture warrior who was fed up with racial mixing and the social degradation of pluralism? "We have to stop these Jews and the Jewish sects from multiplying and diluting our pure Roman magnificence!" Of course, no one thought to limit the ravenous, insatiable conquest which created the Empire and all the wealth which it accrued. It is also entirely possible that his only concern is what we read in the text. He was angry at the loss of economic opportunity. In a complex world we sometimes forget that the profit motive is sometimes prophetic.

And what did Paul think of this turn of events? Later in the story he will fall back on his own Roman citizenship though he does not at this point. As intelligent and culturally aware as he was Paul likely understood the convergence of factors which resulted in the prison cell in which he lay and the stocks in which he was fastened. It was not time to bicker and criticize. It was not time to assert the rights which were his, thereby embarrassing the authorities and escalating the emerging contest between the Pagan establishment and the emerging Christian proclamation. There is no record of complaint. Acts describes a quick arrest, impromptu abuse, and perfunctory incarceration. Paul does not make his Roman citizenship an issue until later when the city leaders acted in hypocritical secrecy.

Paul and Silas. Together, yet isolated. Cut off from the colleagues in whose lives they had invested and with whom they had shared seasons of refreshment and encouragement. They were separated as well from the newly gathered group of Christians who, having come to faith in the great Shepherd of the sheep, now found themselves without the immediate under-shepherd through whom they had first heard of their new Lord. The jail was damp. The conditions inhuman. The stocks cramping. Their outlook— faithfully hopeful.

RESPONSIBLE RESOLUTION

The dark and damp has a way of absorbing sound. Is that the breath of another person or the scritch-scratching of a rat? Some cry. Others rave. Still others curse and demean. Yet there in the dark, lonely confines of an undeserved jail cell two sang.

> Acts 16:25 *About midnight Paul and Silas were praying and singing hymns to God, and the prisoners were listening to them," (Acts 16:25 ESV)*

It certainly does not seem like the right response. It would not appear that it would help. Religious "fervor" was what got them tossed in the stocks and locked in the jail in the first place. Why sing when singing only draws attention to all the differences which created the conflict in the first place?

In singing Paul and Silas were turning inward and outward at the same time. Like Jesus in the desert, they knew that the indistinct sound they heard might just be the serpent slinking into their cell to mock them in their misery, undermining and weakening their faith. In hymn and psalm, in prayer and scripture, strength could be found not only to endure pain but also to respond to the scandal-mongering voice of the dragon. Temptation comes in times of plenty and in times of pain. Satan has perfected his techniques throughout the ages so that when opportunity presents itself, he is able to sidle up to us with just the right words of salacious defeatism to make us abandon the faith. His words in jail cells are far different from those he utters in palaces, yet his ultimate objective is the same.

So, Paul and Silas—likely invisible to one another in the darkness of that presumably subterranean prison, separated not by social contract or shame but by encumbering chains and lingering aches and pains incarnated for those around them the heavenly presence in faithful melody. Of course, they sang! What else is there to do? How does one sulk in solitary? Who does one complain to when everyone whose rasping breath you can hear shares in the same fate?

Creating a worshipping community, bringing the heavenly harmony to life in the midst of misery is what believers do! The Judeans singing "by the rivers of Babylon" were not there for the fishing. They had been sent into well-deserved exile because of their continual bent to sin. In that unfolding disaster they began to rediscover their allegiance to the One True God. David sang in a cave hiding from Saul, his best friend's Dad, his own father-in-law, one of his mentors, whom he recognized as the rightfully anointed King. What else can you do, where else can you turn, and who better to address in your misery when all other options seem futile? Even if no one else heard their voices God attended to their worship.

Now, we don't think of what they were doing in that prison cell as congregating. They numbered only two, there were likely, many more. These others did not share their allegiance to Jesus Christ. They had likely not even heard of Jesus until that very night through those very songs. Some may have been Jews. We know that they were not even nascent Christians because, to let the cat out of the bag just a bit, the real revival had not yet started. It was two guys. Two guys isolated in their cell and likely from one another. No allies other than themselves. A captive audience who witnessed firsthand what it means when the body of Jesus is attacked and His people must fall back entirely on faith. Create community. Make Jesus present. Enfold every soul present in the love and incarnate presence of Christ.

In that lonely cell psalms and hymns made Christ incarnate all over again, as psalm and hymn still do whenever the Church faithfully gathers in worship. One must speculate, since we are not told exactly which Psalms, they sang or what the content of the hymn or hymns were. Maybe they sang a song like this one, perhaps you have heard or read these words.

> *5 Have this mind among yourselves, which is yours in Christ Jesus, 6 who, though he was in the form of God, did not count equality with God a thing to be grasped, 7 but emptied himself, by taking the form of a servant, being born in the likeness of men. 8 And being found in human form, he humbled himself by becoming obedient to the point of death, even death on a cross. 9 Therefore God has highly exalted him and bestowed on him the name that is above every name, 10 so that at the name of Jesus every knee should bow, in heaven and on earth and under the earth, 11 and every tongue confess that Jesus Christ is Lord, to the glory of God the Father. Philippians 2:5–11 (ESV)*

It is simply not possible for us to know whether this does or does not represent the lyrics to the hymn—the tune of which is equally mysterious. Scholars and academics assert that this famous "kenosis" passage from the Epistle to the Philippians (that is, the Church Paul was in the middle of establishing when the incident we are discussing took place) was most likely a hymn which was already being sung in the churches when Paul used it to address the Philippian congregation. He chose it because it was a familiar, maybe treasured, perhaps theologically formative song to the congregation. If it was, in fact, a hymn already known to the Philippians when Paul included it in the epistle, who taught it to them? I will wait just a moment for you to think and then blurt out the answer. Paul taught them this hymn, and though this is not really the forum for debating with those academics and scholars I mentioned earlier, it is likely that Paul himself composed the lines and taught the song to the Philippian Church while among them. This accounts for what is the theological high point of the epistle. Not that he is giving a new and innovative teaching to them about the need for humility considering the supreme sacrifice of Jesus. Rather he is reminding them of what he has already taught them about Jesus the incarnate Son. Crucified Servant. Resurrected Sovereign. He not only taught that message he embodied it, even when—especially when, singing in a jail cell.

The result of this impromptu worship was something the early Church expected and which we find a little frightening. Kingdom came and Empire shook. Maybe the jailhouse after-action report went something like this:

Centurion: "Just tell us what happened."

Guard: "Well sir, these two guys were singing and all of a sudden it seemed like the whole of whatever God is was right here in the jail."

Centurion: "So, it was an earthquake. We all felt it. What happened then?

Guard: "Well, by Marc Antony's grave I thought I'd really screwed up. Surely the prisoners had escaped! I was ready to do my duty to the Empire and take my own life, but they didn't escape at all! The bossy little bald one who kept correcting the other guys singing said 'Don't do that, silly, we're all here!'"

Centurion: "OK, so you locked the prison, and secured all the prisoners. Then what?" Guard: "Well I took them home, apologized, cleaned them up, listened to what Paul (that was the bald one's name) had to say, and decided that me and mine are going to join up with this guy and learn more about this Jesus. Then I took a special bath."

Centurion: "That'll be all."

Guard: "What else was I supposed to do!? It was like God reached down and shook the whole earth to get my attention!"

It is nice to speculate about what goes unsaid in scripture. What we do know is that Paul and Silas were less alone in that cell than any Roman magistrate ever imagined.

That was not the end of the incident. The magistrates were a little embarrassed to discover that "the bossy little guy" was a Roman citizen. Roman citizens could not be beaten nor jailed without trial. To add insult to embarrassment at sloppy police work they had to escort Paul and Silas out of the jail, discreetly asking them to find another city in which to incarnate the body of Christ.

As we conclude our consideration of Paul and Silas and their momentary, light affliction, let us imagine another conversation, this one with Lydia and her household, the Jailer and his. "Tell us brother Paul, what did you do in jail?" Unable to contain a smile the Jailer blurts out "They sang! They sang and the Empire trembled." (He was kind of excited, new creature in Christ and all.)

"What did you sing about?" "Oh," said Paul, "You know, just a little ditty I've been working on to help folk like you understand better who Jesus is and why He sacrificed so much to take on flesh and save us." "Is it hard to sing?" "Can I learn it on my lyre?" "Teach us! Teach us this song before you go so that we can always remember what happened in Philippi when the Kingdom of God shook up the Empire."

"Well, OK," said Paul. "If you *really* want to encourage one another in Christ, get over yourselves. Learn to love in selfless humility like Jesus loved. Think of others first and stop being so narcissistic, narrow-minded, and needy."

"I'm not sure I could sing that" interjected the jailer. "That's not the song. This is the song . . .

> Think like Jesus
>> Who, forsaking his norm.
> Refusing to grasp
>> and cling to the form.
> Gave it all up, creature to serve.
>> Gave it all up to live and die
>>> He Gave it all up, becoming empty
>>> Gave it all up for you and for me.
> Awaiting the day when "He is Lord! We all cry!

. . . that's sort of the first-draft. You know we were in a dark jail cell. I will polish it up a bit and Luke will help me with the tune.

Maybe I'll send you the final version." Lydia hugged him. The jailer shook his hand and banged him on the back (he was a soldier after all) and both said in one way or another "That will work."

5

On the Rock Alone?

He who stilled storms
Uses storm as His voice
And He strides on the crystalline
waves.

He who walked Galilee's
Hills and ravines.
Abides with the exile
Flockless, alone.

Last of his line who walked
With the Master
He misses His flock
And writes as their pastor.

Either in torture
Or in exile-do pray
In the Master's name
In His Spirit.
On His Day.

A FAMILIAR STORY

ONE OF THE SIGNAL moments of creation, described in the Book of Genesis is the creation of the sea when God seperates the waters above from the waters below. This creative act of the Father's will, spoken into actuality through the dynamic Word was witnessed by no one. There is a corollary to be found in one of the most powerful and liberating visions found in the final book of the Bible. However, at that moment when the sea representing separation sunders no more—at that point there is a witness, in a very real sense, the last witness. A witness who had outlived his peers and been given visions of final salvation and consummation. In John's vision, the sea and all that separates is removed forever so that the redeemed may revel in God's presence eternally singing the song of the Lamb.

He was the right one to see and hear and write about the final triumph of Kingdom over Empire. His companions had suffered. Some more cruelly than others. They had given the full measure of their strength to implement the vision of their Master. Jesus had taught them Himself what it meant to sacrifice everything for the sake of the Kingdom, so they did not hesitate when asked to abandon everything, even the very breath of life, for the sake of following Him.

John had spent his youth on the open water. He had grown up awakened each morning by the chattering of the gulls and slipped to sleep each evening listening to the shaping, slapping, surge of the surf. He had gained strength and experience. Strength from rowing the boat and hoisting the sail. From hauling the nets filled with fish. Counting the catch and cleaning the equipment. Because he and his brother were trusted by their father, they quickly became very good at sailing the boat and finding the shoals of fish. Then they and their younger contemporaries began to take over the business. Peter was always the cleverest at negotiating and cajoling the best price from the buyers and other vendors which lined the docks and beaches around Capernaum. Commerce also required Peter and his partners to learn how to communicate in

Greek. It was not only the political language of the empire it was the commercial language. So in the far-off Galilee of John's youth, it was the language of fishing, bartering, selling, and dealing with the revenuers. Because it was flexible and universal it was the language in which he would write these last letters detailing the final, apocalyptic visions—previewing the eternal victory, and bringing Scripture to a close. John would describe a victory symbolized—at least for him—by the disappearance of the sea as the end of creation was folded back into its beginning.

The humble Galilee—a large lake really—was not the last sea that John would see. As Empire in its many manifestations slowly drove the embryonic church from the land of its birth it went with an uncompromising desire to reproduce. One can only walk so far out of Jerusalem, past Jericho, around Samaria, through the Galilee before it became necessary to wade from the beach and board a vessel leaving the Levant. Sometimes leaving forever.

Peter his old partner, colleague, and competitor on the lake had begun the movement away from Jerusalem. Others followed. Even James, Jesus' brother, authorized men to "go into the world" though they predominantly dealt only with the descendants of Israel. The gospel was well known both in the capital and in the provinces. It was especially strong here in Asia Minor. Here Paul, who was, in John's opinion, rightly called the *Apostle to the Gentiles*, had worked so long and hard to establish the faith first preached along the Sea of Galilee, on the shores of the Adriatic Sea.

From shore to shore, the faith had truly reached the uttermost parts of the earth. A faith first heard on the beaches, and boats on the Galilee now had adherents planted on the shores of nearly every known sea, ocean, lake, and river in the Roman world. The Mediterranean, right in the middle was for all intents and purposes a body of water bounded entirely by the Church. The Adriatic, Aegean, and Black seas were fast becoming Christian lakes. Even the shores of the vast Atlantic and beyond to the frigid stretches of the North Sea there was occasionally heard the voice of followers of Jesus in prayer, song, and proclamation.

He had not known Paul well, but he knew his fruit. Paul, like all visionaries always had more to say than audiences could hear. He had a passion which few could hope to match. Yet he had surrounded himself with a vigorous community of young men and women that he was able to shape and mold into an effective team in pursuit of the unified goal of converting the empire. The work was not yet complete—but an enormous harvest had been brought into the storehouse of the Kingdom. John knew some of that fruit intimately, at first-hand, and by name. He knew what Paul had taught and how well he had taught it because the people that he himself missed so dearly right now had been discipled, converted, and prepared by Paul and his large, capable team. They had learned the story of Jesus. They had learned how Jesus taught His earliest followers to read the Scriptures in a revolutionary way. They had been focused on what was required of them as subjects of the Kingdom in a world devotedly focused on the ends of Empire.

And they knew him! When he emigrated to the region around Ephesus, he expected to be received by the Churches but not recognized! They relished the stories he told of His own time with the Master. Those blessed times seemed so long ago now. So many of his friends had joined the "great cloud of witnesses". In continuing to preach, and write, and teach, he connected the beginning with the present and prepared the entire Church for the future. The last of those who first followed the Master. A final witness. John in Asia was a fitting benediction to the first generation. He added to the treasures of Gospel story, wrote letters, led the Church, and opposed false teachers.

Asia Minor attracted cults, sects, gurus, and mystery religions of all kinds. In many ways it had become the cultural heart of the empire. What took root in West Asia soon found its way throughout the entire Roman world. Some of those new and emerging movements saw the Church as natural competition for both converts and wealth. Consequently, there was always a need for clear teaching, faithful exegesis, and accurate preaching. Some of these movements discovered that the best approach to dealing with the Church of Jesus was to try and meld the teaching of Jesus into whatever spiritual tonic you were peddling. Syncretism was the lynchpin of pagan thought! Compromise worked just as well as competition. You could never have too many gods!

And beyond pure religion there were philosophical disciplines and schools which were early blended with Christian doctrine to form a new, knowledge-based cult deriving power and influence, not from the message of Jesus but from a repackaged appeal to self-deification. They treasured their secrets: hidden documents, mysterious rituals, maybe even secret hand-shakes and signs. John opposed these "know-it-alls"[1] as they called themselves because Jesus alone was the way, the truth, and the life. He remembered those words and used them often, spoken as they were so long ago by the Master Himself.

He was firm and focused, formidable in dispute—but no longer (to recall the nickname the Master had given he and his brother) a son of thunder. As he got older and further away from the land of his youth and his first overly zealous adherence to the message of Jesus, he realized more and more that the power was in the way that Jesus' word mediated life changing power. You cannot change someone's life when you are more interested in punishing them. He chuckled remembering when he and little Jimmy, his brother, suggested that Jesus wipe out villages who resisted. Now, after all those years, some of those very villages had flourishing churches. These days his favorite command of the Master, which he repeated as often as he could to as many congregations which would pause long enough to hear an old man out? Love. His own constant refrain in dealing with both the faithful and the fallen? *Love one another.* But now, he was here. They were there. And the churches would have to negotiate a treacherous time by themselves guided by words he could write and that they could read but which they could not hear, nor feel. Here he was at his age, after all he had experienced; alone.

---

1. That is really what the mysterious Gnostics were. Secretive know-it-alls who thought that the way to spiritual power was to be found in secretive rites and an air of superiority.

He did not deserve to be here by himself. He was not really in any shape to subsist in the barrenness of a penal colony. He was not personally offended at the idea of persecution. He was in Ephesus because of the persecution which drove him first from Jerusalem then broader Palestine, finally far away from the Levant. He was not the first, not the last, not the only. Yet, it did seem that he was likely the oldest.

Persecution had been there from before the beginning. What were the stubborn questions Jesus Himself answered during the days of His ministry but probing for weakness or waffling on what was acceptable to the Jerusalem elite and the Pharisaic legalists? He always answered well. He always carried the debate. So, they eventually killed Him. And though Jesus conquered death, He understood and taught the Church, even when it was His small band of disciples "If they came after me . . . they're coming after you too."

Opposition had been there almost from that first Pentecost. He and the others answering all those questions, dodging all those accusations, negotiating all those crises. As arduous as it was this process had helped the Church to define its doctrine and practice more clearly in a fast-moving world. John saw many of his friends and companions die. He was still in Jerusalem himself when James his brother, was martyred. He had suffered and was suffering—yet not as fully as some had. It would have been easier had he been hung, or stoned, or beaten, or beheaded. He would have closed his eyes in this world to fall finally and fully back into the arms of Jesus. Now, he woke every morning sleeping on a hard mattress in a place rightly described as a rock by everyone who had heard about it.

Having firmly established his life on the Rock of Ages, he stood on a rock of isolation looking longingly east to the little flock which still needed the thundering, loving kindness of the last remaining human soul who had walked with Jesus. John looked forward with hope. He looked backward with fondness for what Jesus had accomplished through he and his companion-disciples. When they had first been called by Jesus each had doubts about all the others. During the time of ministry Jesus let them ask silly questions, nurture petty rivalries, and perform small ministry tasks. After the defection of Judas and the denial of Peter everyone finally understood the enormity of what Jesus had in mind, the specificity of purpose it would take, and the identity of the group He would use to change the world. Yes, they had all grown up quickly and became capable most fully when the Spirit had come upon them that Pentecost so long ago.

Now, here on Patmos he saw a vision. He heard a voice. Here in exile, he was entrusted a vital vantage point from which to understand the whole massive story of God's redemptive quest for humanity. Everything told Him by Jesus then and there on Patmos revolved around the essential truth that history's central act was the crucifixion/glorification of Jesus. Everything before was prelude. Everything after postlude. History might take its twists and turns. We human creatures will always stumble forward one step only to trip and fall back two. History is messy and the fall is ever present for Adam's children, created in the perfect image of God yet marred by the narcissistic disobedience of Adam.

The book of Revelation is comically grotesque, filled with exaggerated emblems of Empire and the evil of the Serpent. John wrote this way, with apocalyptic urgency, not because he was insane or to calm our fears or to inflame our passions. He wrote this way because to some extent human history is itself a form of madness and the vibrant images can oddly, serve to at least calm our fear a bit, if it cannot assuage it entirely. Think of the Book of Revelation as a cartoon depicting the futile efforts of Empire to undermine, attack, belittle, horrify, hamstring, and halt the unending march of God toward the redeemed consummation of His creation. Cartoons are designed to exaggerate, simplify, and soften matters too serious for children to yet process. Children understand that there is more than meets the eye. They know there is a joke even when they do not "get it." Because Apocalyptic is an a-historical and non-literal genre, it is also non-threatening. Apocalyptic enables beleaguered Christians to learn how to process abstract information without being terrified by it. Apocalyptic helps the Church, then and now, to see the whole history of God's work in Jesus as complete and inevitable; particularly when the beast of Empire confronts the Kingdom of the Lamb. In this case the truth about Empire—is a comic opera. Satan and all those he has deluded; the ever-expansive evil of Empire, rants and raves and seeks to destroy as the redeemed celebrate and sing the song of the Lamb.

There is no more dramatic book in the Bible than this book. Revelation begins with Jesus giving John an encouraging vison of the ultimate victory. The victory of Kingdom over Empire. The victory of Word over confusion. The victory of light over darkness. The victory of presence over exile. In many ways it is the same story we have been considering since I began writing these words and you began reading them. We humans are in some way, despite our strengths and tremendous grasp of our own place in the world, alone. Ours is the solitude of a long slow trek to a death we need not experience but which, for prides sake, we pursue with the vigor of serpent-inspired vanity. All that drama which pours into the book of Revelation was experienced by one man alone with God. Maybe John in his exile should be a model for how we understand the enforced distance between us? In Revelation John testifies that when you are worshipping the God of all creation. You are never truly alone.

I cannot think of a better place for us to finish our trips into the "desert". I can think of no better voice to hear. This is the place to end our time with the lonely and isolated in the New Testament. These stories of patience have the power to instruct us if we have ears to listen and wisdom to assimilate their lessons We think of them as stories of exile, temptation, and adversity. The terms change while the implications are largely the same. Their stories should inform and qualify our still unfolding story. The twenty-first century story of the socially distanced, the quarantined, the sequestered. We are not the first. We are not the last. We are not the only. There is hope in our exile, there is God's presence in our solitude.

We end here not only because it is the end of the book, but because the visions of John which have been ever true since he first saw them remind us that life finds us acting out a parable. A parable which John surely heard from the lips of Jesus; the parable of the weeds. This parable reminds us that in our world there is good and bad. Each grows intermingled with the other. Though we often feel morally compelled to uproot the weeds lest they corrupt the crop, God in His wisdom has determined that to do so is unnecessary, even reckless. In the end the harvest will sort things out. Until that time, we must be faithful. Until then we must be patient. Until then we must be determined. Till the end we must continue with the Mission. Too often our best intentions, even when they are faith-driven, lack patience. John's account of the Revelation of Jesus Christ is often misunderstood and misapplied by turning it into something it is not. It was a word of hope proclaimed to a persecuted Church ministering in a hostile empire. The images often considered frightening and outrageous are designed to teach courage and patience. Jesus reveals Himself to John who is instructed to teach the Churches regarding faithful witness in the worst of times. Much of the ludicrous and extravagant hype expended in exploiting and explaining the book of Revelation either forgets this purpose or ignores it. Why pass along John's words of hope when you can inflame the fears of the impressionable by confusing symbols with contemporary events?

And among the most egregious omissions? John, the lonely visionary himself! He is shoved aside, and his words of hope and encouragement transformed into "tracts for the times" intended to startle the masses and surprise them into something like repentance. All the while turning the church into a purveyor of secretive insider information. Rather than proclaiming public words of exhortation the Church focuses on moralistic escapism. Rather than proclaiming faith, hope, love, grace, and the redeeming presence of God the Church wags its finger and says "You're gonna get yours!" Rather than a dignified discussion of salvation-history the Church conducts a role-reversing pantomime longingly wishing that the shoe was on the other foot and that Kingdom had political power and influence. A development John would find incongruous and laughable. So, John is ignored and the churches to which he wrote—conjured into pretend abstractions rather than historical congregations involved in a life-and death struggle with a hostile empire bent on eradicating their message and mission.

I have taught and preached from the book of Revelation many times. I have been asked many more times and demurred. It has been my experience that most who ask have already made up their minds about its message and are hoping to involve me in an officially sanctioned process of confirmation bias. I will not participate. I am convinced that the book of Revelation needs to be understood and that its message is about far more than a checklist for the end of time. The Apocalypse unveils all scripture. But like Jesus said, "not everyone has ears wide open." If you ever hope to understand anything of the book of Revelation that understanding will begin with an appreciation for the lonely shepherd who longingly looked across the chaotic sea hoping to provide pastoral encouragement to his endangered flock. The book of Revelation, the vision he saw, and the words which he wrote is that message of hope intended to remind the Church that when seemingly alone on distant shores, experiencing the threat of extermination at the hands of an enraged beast of Empire; the Good Shepherd sees and hears and is walking—even if unseen—among His churches. Once again, the perception that we are alone, whether John on Patmos or his churches, is a snake-breathed illusion, a dragon's tale conceived to crush our spirit. Jesus knows. Jesus sees. He has the keys to the Grave—His and ours.

A DISTURBING DEVELOPMENT

Here's a rough rendition of how John begins his message to the seven mainland churches from which he is sundered . . .

> *Friends, this is John. The good news is I'm alive! The bad news? I've been exiled. The real story—however is what happened last Sunday! I saw and heard the Master again! My old Galilean friend appeared to me—not as in days of old as a rustic traveler—but as the Ancient of Days. I saw Him in all His splendor, and He had an important message for me to send to you based on the visionary conversation*

we had. You need to understand that His conquest of death; despite the efficient approach of you-know-who means that He is our Savior, Sovereign, Eternal Lord, and Judge. So, like I was saying, I was exiled to this rock for standing on the "solid Rock" (always be preaching lads!) but that did not stop me from worshipping, praying, reciting the word—in short, I was doing what the Lord's people, filled with the Lord's Spirit do on the Lord's day-and that is when I saw Him. That is when I heard Him. So, listen up. He's got a few pats on the back, some kicks in the backside, and sadly—some warnings.

For both John and Jesus the ultimate issue, the most disturbing development, was not violence. They were adequately prepared for that eventuality. Jesus' crucifixion set the standard. There had already been many "martyrs."[2] Waves of persecution broke out in various sectors of the Empire for different reasons. In some areas it was the continued animosity of formative Judaism against the earliest followers of Jesus. By this stage of their individual growth into distinct faith communities the Synagogue and the Church had devolved to the level of invective and name calling. In an inflammatory and syncretistic religious environment it was only a matter of time before cat-calling became physical conflict. Paul had participated in such campaigns in the earliest days, prior to his conversion. Afterwards, he had himself experienced both violence and imprisonment. Ultimately his name was added to the list of those who gave their all for the cause of Christ. John's own brother Jimmy (James) was among the first. Then Peter, and James the brother of the Lord . . . and on . . . and on. Yet believers never became jaded, and they never forgot. Soon it became apparent that neither the hermeneutical conflict with synagogue

2. Some terminological clarification. The word "m a r t u r e o" means to bear witness. The noun form signifies someone who "gives witness." The message they bring is "testimony." This sort of reasoning is still evident to this day in our court systems. Martyr, Martyrdom, and their Testimony become technical terms to delineate those who gave the ultimate testimony to the faith—giving their lives. To this day we use the term in the way that evolved in earliest Christianity to describe those who sacrifice themselves for the sake of Christ, His Church, and the message of the Gospel.

nor the institutional violence of Empire worked. Violence did not achieve the ends hoped for. Not only did violence fail—it made things worse. By their faithful example the Martyr Church under pressure still served, still loved, still extended kindness, still lived generously, and still grew. Explosively!

Empire had other tools. For generations the Adversary had been sharing his serpent shaped strategies for undermining and overthrowing God's redemptive purposes. Though he knew for certain that the failure of crucifixion sealed his destiny, he was hell-bent on filling the pit before the end. And humanity for all the gifts given by the Creator, had developed many weaknesses. Like old Jacob from the ancient story, all humanity loped lazily into the future with a limp. Jacob got his by finally getting his hands on God and not letting go. Most other humans came by their limp as an inevitable result of the fall.

Sex worked. Hunger could be exploited in several ways. Starvation and gluttony were means to an end. Sex was particularly effective. Drunkenness was a favorite because it was so entertaining in an endless variety of ways! Violent drunks, funny drunks, maudlin drunks, passed out drunks—oh the fun! Sex never failed. It did not seem to matter how attractive or ugly a man was there always appeared to be some other human person who appealed to them as so overwhelmingly attractive that all other thoughts vanished and all restraints were abandoned. Money. Greed. Sex. Selfishness. Quite an arsenal. And all could be combined and altered and leveraged. To create a cocktail of temptation and possible damnation. So many appetites. So little self-control.

He had, of course offered a sub-set of these temptations to Jesus—who, you will recall, refused. But even his followers, those determined disciples the audacious apostles, and all those persuaded by this new messaging . . . even the most faithful, the most committed were human, were marked by the fall. Walked with that limp. These liabilities could be exploited.

And Empire, the Empire, this Empire was the perfect vehicle not only to threaten but to thrill! Its "peace" was a hoax, but how enormous, how enthralling, how effective it was! The ease with which it deflected attention from the heartless avarice and rapacity which was at its core was simply brilliant. And who wouldn't want a piece of that. With the peace came stability and wealth. And where some became wealthy others became envious! What a perfect environment for chaos! Merchants brought "exotic" materials from the "east" (It's just a direction unless you can make it pejorative or mysterious). Merchants sold slaves. Merchants held "games". Import and export. Exploit and expand. Commerce as ideology. One more arm of the beast rising from the sea. And as those merchants plied their trade across the Mediterranean; the middle-of-the-(Roman)-world-sea, they owed it all to the man on the throne in the eternal city and the genius which kept him there. All that glitters was not gold. But the glittering did help advertise the system, and despite the deception, there was much gold.

And what could not be bought or sold could be foisted on the gullible through superstition. These people worshipped everything. Every single thing. They would believe virtually anything. Though it seemed to be too great of a leap for them to imagine that the only one who deserved their worship could not be objectified, marketed, or managed. Moses had told them. Abraham had known generations before when the whole enterprise of Empire had just been getting off the ground. Yet repeatedly both in the culture addressed by Gods Word and other cultures which seemed forgotten; men, women, slave and free-even children could be seduced with shiny, distracting objects which provoked their desires. Their lust was limitless. Their eyes ever wandering. Their minds easily confused.

It was this juxtaposition of the multifaceted sinfulness common among fallen man and the Imperial impulse to control and commercialize it which presented the pressing need for which Jesus appeared and John wrote.

The tactic was no longer to just beat the Church into submission. The counterproductive tactic of only attacking the Church physically with brute force would be supplemented by other approaches. Seduce it. Tempt it. Give the Church an incentive to combine elements of Gospel with the mysteries. Combine the opulent cults and rituals which promised ecstasy with the "power of Empire" to grant favor. Provide an environment of compromise in addition to coercion. Threaten starvation in an Empire which had plenty. Make it easy for Christians to see themselves as good citizens of the Empire not through attacking them but by expecting them to behave *normally*. Malign them. Marginalize them. Don't strike when words can do just as much harm.

In this emerging environment of all-out attack on the Church hope would come from a resolute commitment to the person of Jesus, the principles of the Gospel, and the priorities of mission. Hope would be lost when the either the attacks of the Empire or the allure of its riches loomed larger than the empty tomb of the Risen one.

RESPONSIBLE RESOLUTION

How do John and his vision of Jesus serve to bring hope to a lonely, persecuted church? How can one exiled man, who appeared to be utterly isolated himself, bring hope to those whose best approach to the unfolding crisis seemed to be hiding? Like all the individuals we have examined in this book, what seems obvious about John and his circumstances is really not as it appears. He was exiled yet in perfect communion with his risen Lord. The solitary confinement, the governmentally enforced social distancing did not have the desired effect. The Roman officials who governed Asia Minor clearly thought that in removing their most significant leader the congregations would scatter and might even be divided. They didn't even need to make John a martyr. They thought that silencing his voice with distance—removing his power by removing his presence would be enough to accomplish their task. They had a plan. It seemed effective. It appeared moderate. They were wrong.

The central reason that their plan went wrong tells us less about John than it tells us about Jesus. They thought Him a man long dead whose voice had been silenced by the cross. If you have followed our web of stories so far you understand how flawed this assumption really was. They presumed that at best John was a misguided mystic, a preacher so taken with his own wit and wisdom that he had come to believe the far-fetched stories he told when these Christians assembled. The other option was that he was simply a madman who would be quickly forgotten once the churches could no longer be enthralled by his gaze, his presence, his performance. What they never considered, what they did not account for, was that John was in communion with the Living Christ. They never considered it a possibility that John's responsible—dare we say revolutionary response—would entail continuing to do and be who Jesus had called him and formed him to be, continuing to do what he had been called to do so many years before. There was no distance too great for someone serving the Risen One.

It is easy to become so caught up in the visions, the images, the picturesque and emblematic portrayal of the battle between Kingdom and Empire that we forget the forgone conclusion of its outcome. When we read the book without considering John's intent, his purpose, and the central message of the book we forfeit the power of its hopeful outlook. Though the book fascinates some and fills others with fear it is seldom proclaimed faithfully because sensationalizing its content is much more marketable than putting it into its proper context and linking its message to the rest of the New Testament. In the same way that the book of Acts is a history of the proclamation of the gospel and that the Epistles are less personal communication than they are expositions of the Gospel, the Revelation of John is simply one more way of telling the story of Jesus; symbolically reconfigured on a cosmic, universal scale.

Because the book of Revelation is read by so many in service of a theological tale which is only remotely related to the Gospel of Jesus Christ it is easy to miss the most important part of the scene I have already paraphrased and which we will consider in detail as the very heart of John the Exile's response to his exile.

First, we need to understand John and his hopeful message as an extension of his prior witness to Jesus.

> 9 *I, John, your brother and partner in the tribulation and the kingdom and the patient endurance that are in Jesus,*

On the Rock Alone?

*was on the island called Patmos on account of the word of
God and the testimony of Jesus. Revelation 1:9 (ESV)*

The threat the empire saw in John was directly related to his role as witness to Jesus. He opens the epistolary portion of the book by identifying himself almost entirely in relational terms. He connects himself to his audience by reminding them that they are brothers and partners. He may be alone on the rock, and they may feel alone without his personal guidance, yet they are still—despite the circumstances—each continuing the trajectory of ministry begun that day when his physical brother and his actual business partners were first called by Jesus to leave their business, ships, servants, and everything else, there along the Galilean beaches. Though visionary and apocalyptic the book of Revelation reinforces, reconceptualizes, and refocuses the same Gospel.

Despite all the changes which the now elderly John had experienced, he still thought of himself in terms of the brotherly love and affectionate companionship he shared with all those who first answered the call to discipleship. John's strategy during his exile when given the chance to encourage his flock—and through them us—was to unify and strengthen what Empire sought to divide and weaken. It is a positive, constructive response to crisis which we would do well to remember, study, and emulate.

During our long year of exile, during our long-suffering pandemic season there has been too much divisiveness. There has been too much distance. Well and good that we remained physically separated. There was no need for the physical reality to be mirrored in our hearts and acted out within the Church(es). In our technically advanced age, with the remarkable variety of communications technologies at our disposal there should have been no conflict, no loss of love, no coldness to our brothers in Christ.

Regardless of the difficulties of the times in which we live, the followers of Jesus are always united by our filial bond to one another and the responsibilities of witness. John did not see Patmos as a vacation spot or himself as Empire's vanquished adversary but as a ministry opportunity. How have we viewed our Patmos? Did we prepare ourselves for the next season of ministry or did we pout longingly for those things we missed, selfishly seeking to keep a control which we never really had? That is the thinking not of Patmos but of paradise lost. That is the thinking of our first parents who chose to take what was not theirs hoping to find in knowledge a wisdom only granted by time and fellowship with God. We have allowed Empire to dominate our thoughts during this season. We have sulked when we could have served. We became dejected when we could have encouraged. We sat on the rock and stared at the sea forgetting that the one who made the sea also walked upon it. John thought first and always in terms of ministry. John thought about the message he preached and the testimony he bore regarding Jesus. That is what he taught the churches when he was present, and now that Jesus had come to him in vision that was the heart of the message he preached in his absence. Maybe it is time for the Church, for each of us as individual Christians to remember that our calling demands that we take up our cross, lose our life, and follow Jesus. Has there ever been a better time to refine our walk than now? Has there ever been a better environment to relinquish what holds us back? When will we ever again experience a cultural solitude enabling us to reconfigure our lives?

The second emphasis at the heart of John's responsible resolution of his exile is worship.

> [10] *I was in the Spirit on the Lord's day, and I heard behind me a loud voice like a trumpet Revelation 1:10 (ESV)*

Instead of initiating his message to his churches with a diatribe against those who had exiled, insulted, or injured him, rather than complaining about the ill-treatment, loneliness, and bad food he began his message to the Asian churches with a reminder that God's kingdom people are expected to conduct themselves as citizens of that kingdom even during the most trying of circumstances. He was in God's Spirit which is to say that he was attentive to the prompting and leading of God's indwelling presence in his life. It would be easy for him; it would be far easier for any of us in times of duress to become disillusioned and abandon the purpose for which we are called. In crisis, Christian people worship. Christian people know that God will continue to honor their faithfulness as we honor His. God's Church knows that throughout history, the way of faith has been marked with discouraging circumstances. The Church knows that we grow stronger when we worship, pray, proclaim, and express the gospel right through those circumstances. Rather than despair, God's people respond with devotion.

Here is an important message not only to the seven Churches John addresses directly in the Book of Revelation but to those of us who make up the current universal Church. The Church is stressed by circumstances beyond our control, circumstances which have isolated us and separated us from the common elements of our life together. John's message is that those common things, those unifying bonds of faithfulness and love and hope and encouragement and thankfulness still exist during the crisis circumstances which face us. It is our joyful responsibility to explain God's presence in our time; to proclaim His Lordship, exalt His name. The Gospel has not ceased to be the Gospel, the Bible is still authoritative, and Jesus is still Lord. Social distancing, isolation, quarantine, masks and mandates; these are circumstances, these are context. They need not define us. We need not cower in fear when we face the unknown because the Jesus who called us, the Christ who suffered for us, the Lord who reigns over us continues to move within us—individually and corporately even when we are separated.

John could not do anything about his exile. His condition was proscribed for him by others. Circumstance is context, but context need not be destiny. The body of Christ has always existed in a context typified either by neglect or hostility. Sometimes both at the same time! We have become complacent. We have become accustomed to comfort when most of our ancestors expected to live their entire life as outcasts from society.

So, John the witness to Jesus—continued to testify—telling the story of Jesus, his sacrificial love and all-conquering resurrection. John, who learned from Jesus Himself the nature of true worship:

> [23] *But the hour is coming, and is now here, when the true worshipers will worship the Father in spirit and truth, for*

the Father is seeking such people to worship him. John 4:23
(ESV)

John does not lecture those who felt isolated and alienated he simply reminded them that their fears of being left alone were a delusion best disabused by continued worship and devotion. He did not promise that through worship and witness things would "get better" because John was wise enough and had walked the way of the cross long enough to know that the goal was never comfort in or acceptance by the world. Rather, he knew that the task of the Church is to be faithful to the call of Jesus to be disciples. Our responsibility is to bear true allegiance to Jesus by reminding the Empire that physical isolation does not hamper our voice or diminish our vision. John worships and invites them to worship. John tells them the story of Jesus. He tells it in a way more visionary, vibrant, and victorious than seemed possible while suffering persecution and exile. He knew that the Master knew the whole story. How it began. How it would end.

Some may wonder how John's circumstances are analogous to our own. What can we learn from the churches of Asia Minor and the message John sent them? Isn't there something more profound? Isn't there something cosmic, something otherworldly? Isn't there something earth-shattering, grand, and climactic? That's it. John teaches his churches, then and now, that in bending the knee in worship and lifting our voices in praise we are faithfully doing our part to bring the "kingdom come" in our time and place. Does proclaiming the Word and telling the story of Jesus really communicate hope to a world raged by pandemic, distanced by disease, challenged by crisis, and wracked with inequality? It did then. It has throughout history. It can now. The problem is not the virtue of John's solution but our lack of imagination in vigorously applying it.

I know that some reading these words will find fault with me for having missed a signal opportunity to delve deeply into the book of Revelation to find other more scintillating, exciting answers to our current situation than: 1. Witness, 2. Worship. Surely there is more to it than that! We have suffered a year of isolation!

Isn't it at least theoretically possible that vaccines are a modem "mark of the beast? What about all the images of conquest, and chaos, and "hey you've not mentioned Armageddon!"

John's message was both to the Church universal and individual congregation's in particular, historical circumstances. We are one circumstantial instance, one brief snapshot of that much larger assemblage of the Saints; those who have gone before and those to come. To read the Bible as if it were only intended for our time and place and speaks most eloquently to our circumstances is the height of hubris. The very sort of hubris which has made the pandemic worse. It is our pride that has prolonged our painful separation. It is our vanity which has clouded our judgement and convinced us that this cannot be happening to us. The very last thing we need is self-centered readings of any part of God's Word—particularly the Book of Revelation—which only inflame and increase the hubris, pride, and vanity which faith must first crush if Christ is to have His way with us.

Maybe we needed the pandemic to strip away the strengths which had become weakness. Perhaps it was time for some of us to spend quality time away from others, not for narcissistic indulgence but for prayer. Maybe we needed to make all of those sacrifices we shared during virtual worship to remember how to appreciate the real thing. Maybe we needed to mourn so that we could truly celebrate.

Everyone knows that John ends his visionary message by describing the New Heavens and the New Earth; realities only possible because our Lord promises that He is making all things new. It is easy to miss what, for John, must have brought closure to his journey.

From his youth until he responded to Jesus' call, the sea had, for John, represented separation. Not only symbolically but in actuality. When he was working at sea he was separated from his loved ones, excepting those who were in the boat with him. He likely did not romanticize the sea as some do. It was a place of labor. It was a place of chaos and potential death. For John, the sea was his familiar and dangerous workplace.

Now after all those passing years things had not changed all that much. The sea still imposed itself upon cherished relationships. The sea separated him from those he loved. The sea kept him from personal contact with Christians he had led to faith and those who he had nourished and nurtured and nudged into leadership.

John was given the vision, shared the hopeful message, and cherished the thought. The distance will be closed like the scattering of fog in the breaking sunlight. Our isolation will be lost in emerging fellowship. Creation itself will be eluded into eternity. The sea will be no more.

Epilogue: Processing Pandemics

THE PANDEMIC AT LEAST seems to be abating. There will still be difficult issues confronting the Church as we bring this difficult year to a close. The reflections, after-action reports, memoirs, and post-mortems are beginning to roll in. Like this book you are soon to finish. One of the issues that will need to be addressed as this crisis ends and as we consider what to do when we encounter the inevitable *next time*, is the notion of exceptionalism. I will not say American exceptionalism because though we Americans might be better at the conception of national exceptionalism, we are, to use this phrase once again: *not the first, not the last, and not the only* people to feel secure in their exceptionalism. It is tempting to primarily view this crisis in ideological terms. As[1] a pastor-theologian tasked with the regular study and proclamation of Scripture it has been my intent in this book to nudge the Church away from the ever-satisfying indulgence of injured pride.

Ideologies rise and fall very quickly. Long after the true ideologues have had their say and the intellectual cause for which they

---

1. I recognize that in the USA the impact of the pandemic is disproportionately felt in communities of color. It is for others to tell that tale. There are many levels of hubris which need to be addressed. As a pastor-theologian my bailiwick is applying biblical theological reasoning to this problem. To that end my concern has been to highlight how chronological snobbery has defined the exceptionalism which has vaulted the entire world . . . every single nation-state, into a catastrophe. The driving force has been fallen humanity basically making a rude gesture at what it assumes is a largely benevolent, controllable, impersonal "nature" only to find out that "IT" *can* happen to us, now, here. Oops.

campaigned has been cast upon the ash-heap of history, shadow conspirators breathe new life into discarded ideas hoping to gain renown on the coat-tails of the creative. Attacking ideologies is like shooting ducks in a circus arcade. It is easier than shooting real ducks because the ducks can't fly away and the stakes themselves are children's amusements.

In the real world contest between Kingdom and Empire we need to be crystal clear about what is at stake. Others will need to say wise and considered things about how nations, and states, and political entities have weathered this storm. My Church is filled with people. Fallen people. Redeemed people. People who know Jesus well and people who are just coming to know Him. The task of the Church is to always be the Church even when—particularly when—the cultural winds she faces seek to blow her off course.

I have tried to reframe Biblical stories in such a way that we can learn a specific lesson from them. Lonely isolation is a part of the fall. When we experience it as believers it should be a reminder of how things were prior to our absorption into the broader body of Christ.

Understanding and applying Scripture is hard. It is far easier to moralize. It is far easier to allegorize. It is still easier to use the Scripture as a launching point from which hobby horses are ridden and the sacred cow of others are sacrificed. I have tried to avoid those extremes. This is not that. Now is not then.

The hermeneutical process has been described as both a spiral and an intersection of two horizons. While each of those sentiments has been formative in my own growth as a student and preacher of scripture it has been my experience that even those classic descriptions are simplifications.

In this case, perhaps the difference in time, the distance in space, and the distinction in circumstances between the Biblical text and our own time is beneficial. The first century is not like ours. We are not in the classical era in the Middle East. We are mostly not poor or marginalized.[2] So our task is, has been and

---

2. I state this as a non-absolute because, of course, circumstance is always relative. However, starving in the ancient world and starving in 21c USA are

always shall be applying the timeless truth of the scriptures in ever-evolving contexts. The speed at which context evolves, has of course, accelerated in the last 150 years. It is still not clear whether this rapid pace of change is evolution or devolution. This cannot be determined within the processes of history but is a part of the after-action report. That report will, of course, be of God's making. The closing of an epoch or episode does give us a preliminary peek at the success or failure of our contemporary culture. What is it accomplishing and where it is going? An important part of a disciplined, generous understanding of history is knowing exactly when to make a preliminary attempt at understanding the recent past. Perhaps we will look back and in a Churchillian moment of rhetorical grandeur we will be able to pronounce 2020 "their finest hour." Maybe. Maybe not. Don't hold your breath. Keep your head down, pray furiously, believe whole heartedly and walk by faith; not sight.

Faithfulness transcends context though it is always embedded within and expressed within specificity. That should be the first lesson in Discipleship 101. Sadly, it is not. Too often the Bible is taught as if it is magical. Say these words. Invoke this or that hero from the past and "presto!" All is right. Simply reading these stories, just going through the process of actively reading these texts should make it abundantly clear that it is simply not that easy.

- Our time does not determine who we are, but it does locate us.

- The Space we occupy does not limit our horizon, but it does limit our field of action.

- Circumstance can and does change. Often that change is produced by those of us embedded in the circumstance in question.

Let me repeat, what in my mind is a signal word in our time together. The word for the issue at hand is specificity. How do we

---

not the same thing. The impoverished in Palestine or Philippi did not Tweet their need for food, nor was there local reporting. Again; applying scripture requires a supple mind as we connect eras and fill in the analogical gaps.

take a Bible Story which happened then and there under a clear set of conditions; translate it into generalized propositions, and then re-apply it into new, quite different specific times and places. That is the most essential task of preaching. That is the exegetical lodestone. That is the whole point of reading, struggling with, interpreting, exegeting, preaching, teaching and ultimately, living these stories.

If we are to process this set of quarantine conditions, if we are to draw up a prospectus of pandemic outcomes, we need to be fluent in the language of Biblical faith and flexible in our appreciation of what goes on in Biblical stories. We must be increasingly creative in our application of the old, old story in new and different contexts. As the culture becomes more self-centered and the church more oppositional, creative engagement with the Word, the world and the worshipping community will be essential in bringing the faithful to their senses and the faithless to their knees.

That is what I have tried to do here. These stories, taken from the life of Christ and the embryonic Church are not just the same story told from different perspectives. This work is not like exegeting synoptic parallels from the Gospels. There are significant differences between the stories we have shared. The thread that connects these stories, that unifies these passages is not a thick one and it is certainly not one I had noticed until the extenuating circumstances of plague opened my eyes.

Being alone can be isolation. Being alone can be solitude. Being alone can mean loneliness. Being alone can mean perspective. In examining these episodes from the New Testament and approaching them with a synthetic rather than a generic unity my hope is to help disciples, and maybe even a few who are not, to find a peace that only comes when we reduce the time, space, and circumstantial conditions between the Word to which we listen and the World in which we live.

Another possible way of describing this experience is that it is bounded. Each of us has a "here." Each of us lives with a "them." All of us have "now". These boundaries bleed into each other. I am sharing my time and place and people with the time, place, and people of other individuals. We work together, worship together, attend events together. Some of us share grandchildren, some of us share hobbies and phobias. Virtually every human person shares our bounded experience with others, yet for each; our experience is not limitless. Many of us in the Postmodern West have simply forgotten that the horizon plays tricks on our eyes and that for some activities the sky really is the limit. When you close your eyes tonight even as you lay next to your wife you will be alone. Alone in your unconscious mind, alone in your dreams. Just you and God.

Christian faith helps individuals process their bounded stories by gathering and telling them in the company of others who share their basic outlook on life. We may not know what you know or see all that you see but our experiences are analogous enough that we can at least peek over the boundaries that define our lives and share what we have seen of the *times* in which we live, the *spaces* we occupy and the *circumstances* which define us.

Jesus stepped into time to redeem it. Jesus stepped into space to sanctify it. Jesus stepped into historical contingency to complete it.

End Matter

I GENERALLY LOOK AT the bibliography of a book first. It is often a reliable guide to where the author intends to take you. I particularly like authors who put the bibliography up front. I've produced some materials for lectures which use this format. My favorite kind of bibliography (what kind of a person has an ontology for bibliographies?) is annotated. I like for the researcher to give me an idea of what he or she thinks of a book. Does he quote it more often in agreement or disagreement? What is the nature of his interaction with the book? Did he like it? Not every significant book is likable or enjoyable. Some of the most important books a person can read, particularly when dealing with Biblical subjects, are dense, obtuse, even, boring. Generally then, bibliography first! It's just an attempt to do unto others as I really like to have done for me.

Yet here, I've produced a work which does not only does not put the bibliography first, but it also doesn't have one at all. I feel that this deserves some explanation which, if you have stayed with me thus far, I trust you will endure.

The story I have written did not emerge from a well-thought out bibliographic starting point. For me at least, this is odd and a little difficult. Generally, when conceiving of a sermon series I start with an inventory of my available tools. What I own, what I need to get, and where I want to focus. At the time this book was conceived and written I was preaching from Matthew's Gospel. That study informs a great deal of what is written here. My current Matthew Bibliography is 14 pages. I don't quote from any of those works so it is hardly appropriate to include them. Just because you are wet does not mean you were taking a bath. Though deeply immersed in Matthew, this is not technically (or otherwise) a Gospel study. It may have dampened me a bit, but it did not really impact this work. Last year, at the very beginning of the pandemic I was preaching from Luke. During 2020 I preached from the Acts of the Apostles, some Old Testament passages, and Romans. There were also occasions when, due to the unfolding crises around us, I diverged from my plan and spoke directly to specific issues. I was not knowingly impacted by those studies either. So, to summarize. There is no direct bibliographical path from what I was studying in the eighteen months prior to preparing this manuscript to what you now hold in your hands. To have appended a bibliography would have been pretentious and pointless.

That brings us to citations. There really aren't any. True, there are a few footnotes, but they are really explanatory more than anything else-often nothing more than asides. While I believe that well-researched exegetical work in the scriptures is entrusted to the preaching ministry and teaching office of the Church, I am not certain that what I have written here, in the form in which it is written could be preached. So, for those of you looking for a couple of quick-kill sermons, sorry.

This work then, is not study nor sermon nor exposition. I know that authors are not generally tasked with providing genre-classification for their own works but perhaps this explanation will help future reviewers and/or librarians.

This is an expository reflection. I doubt if anyone asked Pascal about the sources of His *Pensées* or made snarky comments about the lack of proper academic apparatus. It was philosophical, but not a work of philosophy. It was spiritual but not specifically devotional. It spoke to that difficult to define intersection between heart and mind that defies any specific categorization but clarifies many categories. It was a reflection. It was one man's attempt to make sense of his context taking advantage of the entire breadth and depth of his educational and spiritual formation.

That, in part, is what I try to do here. I'm not saying I'm Blaise Pascal. I'm not even the guy to determine whether I've pulled off what I've tried. I'm just a pastor-scholar who has sought to provide a Biblically sound, culturally relevant, spiritually focused reflection on a narcissistic world raged by plague and caged by pandemic. When you've lived as much of it as I have maybe, perhaps, that is all the citation needed.